A SIMPLE GUIDE TO IMMUNITY: ENHANCED REVISED EDITION

A SIMPLE GUIDE TO IMMUNITY: ENHANCED REVISED EDITION

A HOLISTIC GUIDE TO EFFECTIVE AND ALTERNATIVE PROTOCOLS FOR SUPERB IMMUNITY, AUTOIMMUNE DISORDERS INCLUDING CANCER, USING HERBS, NUTRITION, SUPPLEMENTS AND MIND/BODY/SPIRIT CONNECTIVITY

Sarah Zitin

ISBN: 1517210496
ISBN 13: 9781517210496
Library of Congress Control Number: 20353
CreateSpace Independent Publishing Platform
North Charleston, South Carolina

ACKNOWLEDGEMENTS

I want to take this opportunity to thank everyone who made this book possible: the team at Createspace, who worked tirelessly to put my words, vision and heart on paper. To my family, without whose love and support I may not have survived, to my parents, Ellie and Sam Zitin, who gave me the foundation, wisdom and values to understand the meaning of social justice and caring for others, to my friends, who have loyally and without hesitation been in my life for many years- at least, most of you. To my teachers in high school, who always made me feel special, to my teachers at Northwestern University who gave me knowledge and a voice of my own, to The Institute of Chinese Herbology in Berkeley, who gave me the tools of my trade, to The Jaffe Institute of Medical and Spiritual Healing, who taught me about self-love and service to others, to everyone in my life who have impacted me in some way, I give heartfelt acknowledgement, appreciation and gratitude.

Life has been my biggest teacher, and all of the experiences that have influenced me. I am the product of everything around me, and I've drawn my strength, compassion, passion, education and information from it.

I would especially like to thank those of you who literally made this book possible:

Adrienne Kessler, for her generosity and love, my sister, Nura Laird, who is my champion and teacher, my niece, Kamela Laird, my other niece, Rachel Zitin, my cousin, Barry Zitin, Janet Wood, Renji Philip, Jenny Ingersol, Terri Weiss, Chris Pellechi, Aneeth Rajan, Valeri Ross, Elizabeth Wu and Donna Deussen. You all have shown me your love and loyalty in more ways than one, and I love you all from the bottom of my heart.

TABLE OF CONTENTS

Acknowledgements · v
Introduction · ix
Chapter 1   Environmental Toxins and Immunity · · · · · · · · · 1
Chapter 2   Candida: The Silent Enemy · · · · · · · · · · · · · · · 12
Chapter 3   Detoxification · 32
Chapter 4   Personal Triumphs Over Autoimmune
             Disorders · 43
Chapter 5   Cancer: Uncommon Protocols, Nutrition,
             Herbs and Supplements · · · · · · · · · · · · · · · · · 77
Chapter 6   Autoimmune Disorders, Symptoms and
             Treatments ·119
Chapter 7   Immune Support Protocols · · · · · · · · · · · · · · · 134
Chapter 8   Chinese Herbs and their Functions · · · · · · · · · · ·152
Chapter 9   Home Remedies for Immune-Related
             Conditions · 166
Chapter 10   Recipes for Healing · · · · · · · · · · · · · · · · · · ·178
             Epilogue · 199
             Author's Note · 201
             Glossary · 203
             About the Author · 225
             Bibliography · 227
             Online Stores for Herbs, Supplements and
             Nutrition · 233

INTRODUCTION

I am writing this book from a place deep in my heart, where I yearn to educate and inform as many of you as I can. My desire to encourage and impart hope, knowledge, and inspiration is compelling and profound.

I have witnessed a great deal of suffering in my lifetime—that of my family, intimate friends and loved ones, and in the world. It has impacted my heart, soul, and spirit in such an extraordinary way that I am driven to write this book with the hope that I can, even in some small way, end the suffering of people around the world.

I, too, suffered from an autoimmune disorder many years ago. My illness inspired my search for answers, knowledge, practitioners, and anyone or anything that could heal me. Desperation was a palpable motive. I, like many of you, endured sleepless nights, pain, discomfort, exhaustion, frustration, and the kind of soul-stealing anguish that makes living a miserable experience.

Although my life was seriously derailed during childhood, which greatly contributed to my weakened immune system, a glimmer inside of me understood that my illness was a wake-up call, and that my purpose in life was to heal others. It ultimately guided me towards my true passion and vocation. I grew to understand that I needed to be a healer and a conduit for natural, alternative healing.

With this in mind, I began a passionate mission to heal myself, and persisted until I found what I needed. For too many years, I had gone from one doctor to another, only to be told there was nothing wrong with me, that I just needed rest and lots of fluids.

Eventually, that mantra became unacceptable. Clearly, something was wrong, and after so many misleading evaluations, I was compelled to become my own advocate, and embarked on a journey to get help.

My symptoms were like many of yours who suffer from autoimmune disorders: extreme fatigue, depression, frustration, anxiety, swollen glands, fever, muscles aches, and dehydration. They appeared and disappeared periodically. I seemed to feel very ill for no reason, after which I would feel well for no apparent reason.

One very significant and consistent symptom was stress. I tend toward extremes of anxiety, which was a constant companion along with the stress it induced. However, good things came out of bad times, and they pushed me to the next level, as pain and suffering often do.

I say this not to depress you or engage in negativity, but to let those of you know who are ill, that you're not alone, and there is absolutely a way to heal the suffering.

After twenty or so years of being tired of feeling exhausted, the infinite wisdom of universal truth led me to the right people at the right time. I began to work with a chiropractor, whom I finally told how terrible and frustrated I felt. He recommended his own Chinese herbalist, and I connected with him immediately.

For the first time in years, I got an answer: I had Epstein-Barr virus, and it had probably begun when I was nineteen years old (my story is in this book), and had had mononucleosis. They are in the same family of viruses.

I began an herbal treatment protocol, which little by little helped me feel better and better—and hopeful, after so many years of struggling. At the time it felt like a miracle, but in reality, the healing protocol was based on traditional Chinese medicine, which has been available and used successfully for thousands of years.

After many, many months of herbal treatment, detoxification, and changing my diet, mental attitude and spiritual practices, I finally felt well and had no more symptoms or episodes of the virus. That was many, many years ago, and I am gratefully humbled to tell you that I am still well and asymptomatic!

As I mention in this book, if a doctor tells you that your ailment is "incurable" or "untreatable," get a second, third, or even fourth opinion like I did. Natural, alternative, herbal, supplemental, and uncommon treatments have been available for centuries, as have curing cancer and various autoimmune disorders.

This book is written as a labor of love in your honor. I want this book to represent your "call to action," for all of you to heal, be well, stay well and experience the joy, vitality, freedom, and abundance you deserve. We all deserve the best life has to offer, and this is my offering to you.

Use the information in this book to take care of yourself, and understand that your health is in your hands and in the care of practitioners who know how to "heal" you. Healing happens every day. I've seen and experienced it, firsthand, and it's an inside job based on the body-mind-spirit connection. They are all involved in the process of healing, and the one common denominator is *you*.

Old ideas, habits, thought patterns, practices, and ways of thinking and being in the world that don't serve you must go. Now is the time to create a new paradigm for living.

This book is not about medicine. Clearly, it's about detoxification, natural foods, nutritional supplements, organic herbs, and other noninvasive, nontoxic protocols.

We live in a toxic environment, and many of us are working very hard to change that fact. The best we can do is keep our bodies and minds clean, and manage what we take in—physically, emotionally, mentally, and spiritually.

I invite you to read and enjoy this book, to use it as a guide for daily living, and give it to someone you know who might be suffering. You may even save your life, or that of a loved one!

In love, service, and gratitude,
Sarah Zitin
Certified Chinese Herbalist, Holistic Practitioner, Author

A SIMPLE GUIDE TO IMMUNITY

INTRODUCTION TO IMMUNITY

According to Webster's Dictionary, the definition of "immunity" is as follows:

"In biology, *immunity* is the state of having sufficient biological defenses to avoid infection, disease, or other unwanted biological invasion. It is the capability of the body to resist harmful microbes from entering it. Immunity involves both specific and nonspecific components. The nonspecific components act either as barriers or as eliminators of a wide range of pathogens irrespective of antigenic specificity. Other components of the immune system adapt themselves to each new disease encountered and are able to generate pathogen-specific immunity."

In other words, the health of your immune system determines your ability to offset or adapt to unwanted biological invasions. If you are weak or compromised, you're more susceptible to a host of infections, diseases, and pathogenic (disease-carrying) microbes.

On the contrary, when you're strong and balanced, you're more capable of offsetting pathogens and undesirable complications. That is the goal, of course—to discover and implement ways in which to have and maintain good health.

In this book I give straightforward and manageable information on how to keep your immune system healthy while avoiding illness and autoimmune disorders. There are chapters on various topics regarding immunity, detoxification, toxins in the environment, candida, cancer, autoimmune disorders, protocols utilizing foods, herbs, supplements, recipes for immunity, and a guide to various online resources for the best quality supplements and herbs.

Did you know that autoimmune disorders have increased exponentially at alarming rates in the past twenty years? This daunting statistic is due to exposure and vulnerability to environmental pollutants, GMO food sources, antibiotics, medications, diets and heavy metal toxins, to which we are exposed daily.

We inhale and ingest so many different kinds of toxins, chemicals, and pollutants—both in and outside of our homes—that it's a challenge to even identify them all. They are found in food, water, air, and earth, and unfortunately, many of them are invisible.

In the interest of health and well-being, it's important to identify and understand the differences between the choices you can make and those you can't. You can't control the environment, for the most part, and you might not have much of a voice in how technology affects you. Yet you can control where you choose to live, what foods you eat, the products you use, and your understanding of how it all affects you.

Particularly if you live in a large city almost anywhere in the world, you're exposed to many environmental toxins. Industrialization has a premium on our lives. In smaller or rural communities, the majority of the population has a better chance at good health, due to reduced numbers of industrial factories.

The lifestyle you choose has great significance in the prognosis of your health. This book is your toolbox, a resource by which you can learn, become informed, and gain awareness of ways to support your immunity.

Western medical practices certainly play an important role in our lives. Treatments and care are mostly palliative, enabling a patient to feel comfortable. Western medicine is an invaluable method for treating pain and discomfort, but more often than not, isn't curative.

Holistic, alternative medicine, on the other hand, which includes detoxification, diet, supplements, herbs, and uncommon protocols, are a more organic, natural and sustaining way to heal the core, or root, of many health problems. In holistic medicine, the core issue of any disease must be addressed before beginning any treatment.

We live within a system, however, that appears to be more focused on medicine-for-profit, which is fostered by large pharmaceutical companies, the US Food and Drug Administration and The American Medical Association. We're constantly besieged by misinformation about medications, food, water, the environment, and the effects they have on our bodies. Advertising, commercials, billboards, and other avenues of promoting products are ubiquitous, suggesting what we should buy, what is good for us, and how to think. It's your responsibility to inform yourself, to distinguish the truth from the lies.

WHY IS IMMUNITY SO IMPORTANT?

The immune system is the heart and soul of the body—without it we have no life. The immune system comprises the entire body:

- Organs
- Circulatory system
- Muscles
- Bones
- Blood
- Venal system

Since all the body's systems are interdependent, it's important to keep them well-functioning, healthy, and balanced. Balance is, unequivocally, the key to good health!

Where does it start? One place it begins is in the gut, which is the seed, or root of all other body functions. At least eighty percent of immunity lies in the stomach, which means that most diseases begin when the gut, or stomach balance is out of whack. What does the gut do? Under the best of circumstances, it absorbs, filters, processes, excretes, nourishes, supports, and commands the rest of the organs to function. That's why gut health is so crucial to the rest of the body.

The gut contains candida (fungus), bacteria, viruses, parasites, heavy metals, and other invasive toxins. If any or all of these factors reach a tipping point, illness and physical debilitation are sure to follow.

It's important to note that toxins are everywhere, and just because we can't see them, doesn't mean they don't exist. We eat, drink, breathe, and absorb them through our skin, which is the largest organ of the body. All of these offenders finally land in the gut, which then becomes like a toxic dump site.

If we look at the increased numbers of cancer, autism, diabetes, arthritis, heart disease, and other autoimmune disorders on a global level, we can deduce a direct correlation between them and the increase in environmental pollutants and toxins.

In the same way, we are all affected by our mental and spiritual belief system. This is one of the differences between someone who becomes ill, and one who doesn't. If we are genuinely positive and feel empowered in our lives, the less likely we are to succumb to the effects of various pathogens.

How, then, do we learn to live in a way that promotes our own health and wellness? How do we prevent ourselves from being victims of illness and autoimmune disorders? To those of us who are already ill and suffering, this might seem like a daunting, impossible task. Many of us who have experienced chronic and degenerative diseases feel helpless, hopeless, defeated, angry, and exhausted. Chronic illness is a soul-stealer, instigating a cycle of debilitation.

These treatments and protocols are not about magic and miracles, but are based on scientifically researched evidence, in many cases. The concept of alternative, natural medicine is to treat the core problem and eliminate disease at its roots.

Since toxins, inflammation, pathogens, and pollutants are at the core of all illness, particularly in the gut, it's important to begin with a safe and effective detoxification process. The healing journey begins once the body is rid of harmful toxins, at which point the immune system is reorganized and recalibrated for optimum function.

This is only the physiological or biological aspect of healing—in holistic healing practices, it's important to consider the "whole person." Have you ever noticed that when you're angry, upset, irritable, discontent, or just feeling out of sorts, your immune system crashes? Or if you're on a "food roll," eating all kinds of junk and processed foods, you get a sinus infection or feel tired, drained, or emotionally off balance?

Feeling bad or sick has a direct relationship to what you ingest and think about. Foods support either harmony or disharmony, as do the thoughts and messages you send yourself. The good news is, of course, that you create your own reality.

It's interesting to note that if you were to live in a country like New Zealand, where "health foods" don't exist because they're *already* healthful due to regulations and environmental protection, you would simply go to the market, buy food, and be assured of good quality.

This is not the case in the United States, however, because corporate interests currently shift the paradigm of air and water quality, and food regulations. While government agencies are busy de-regulating environmental restrictions and controls, consider paying more attention to what you buy because it's necessary for good health. Unfortunately, reading food labels isn't always the solution, because undesirable chemicals and toxins are sometimes misrepresented or undisclosed.

At the same time, some health food stores and several markets, sell items responsibly and with integrity. As the necessity and demand for more organic and healthful products increase, the food industry is forced to follow suit. As more people become ill with autoimmune disorders of all kinds, they're challenged to discover more resources for all of us to regain our natural state of health.

The purpose and intention of this book is to guide you to the information you need to have a healthy, empowered life. This book is particularly helpful for people who do have health issues and autoimmune disorders. For those of you who are in good health, it's helpful to understand how to maintain it, and what actions to take to help others, if necessary.

For those of you who have health challenges and struggle daily, you're not alone. There is help for you, and many ways in which to heal. There are holistic practitioners, herbalists, integrative medical doctors, naturopaths, and other healers in your neighborhood. Thanks to the Internet, you can find just about anything if you look for it. Welcome to your wonderful healing journey—empower yourself to become your own health advocate and step into your personal magnificence!

CHAPTER 1

ENVIRONMENTAL TOXINS AND IMMUNITY

Whatever happened to the "good old days," when we lived in agrarian societies and grew our own foods? Remember when there were no such things as pesticides, herbicides, heavy metals, toxic chemicals, and genetically modified foods? Technology and modern living are both a blessing and a curse, with the powers to create and destroy. Our biggest advantage is that we all have the ability to know the difference.

Here's an example of the controversial chemical trails, or "chemtrails," you might have observed in the skies all over the country. They look like skywriting or exhaust from plane fuel, but according to many researchers, scientists, and chemists who took time to study and test, these trails are alleged to be toxic chemicals such as mercury, barium, arsenic, strontium, and others. According to the Environmental Protection Agency (EPA), these chemicals might be seeding clouds to change weather patterns for crops and livestock.

If these are toxic chemicals used to seed clouds, which filter down into our environment, our water supply and our crops, it's our responsibility to learn more about them, so we can make informed decisions about how to protect our immunity.

Since our health is essentially in our own hands, we must learn how to nurture and nourish ourselves. The more knowledge and information we have about our personal concerns—health, environment, education, air quality, foods, supplements, herbs, and sustainability on all levels, the better equipped we are to deal with the perils of our time.

In Los Angeles and other major cities, there is an increase in respiratory problems in children and adults. Allergies, sinus infections, pneumonia, bronchitis, respiratory ailments and asthma are on the rise, and people with environmental sensitivities are seriously compromised.

Under the circumstances, it's understandable that people are sicker, feel worse, have more cancer, and often struggle just to maintain their daily lives.

Most frustrating of all is that in spite of the fact that we protest, petition, lead marches, and bring awareness to people and governments about the effects on our food, water, and air, we're not heard in a way that affects change.

Global warming is the quintessential example of environmental pollution. Our habits have created toxic carbons, chemicals from plastic, petrochemicals from cars and industry, dangerous electromagnetic fields, factory fumes, chemical plants, underground mining, fracking, and toxins in the ocean, all of which have an impact on what we eat and breathe.

Although there is controversy about global warming, the consensus seems to be that the damage we've done to our planet has caused a great deal of illness and destruction. Our ecosystem is off balance, and all living things are transforming or dying off. Is this a natural part of our existence? Does the planet ebb and flow like the tides? The sophistication of technology has recalibrated and reconstructed our efforts at sustainability, and natural or not, it's critical that we find solutions to save the planet.

The big corporations seem to win out every time because money talks. Monsanto is the most obvious example. The government has actually sanctioned this conglomerate to consistently create GMO (genetically modified organisms) foods, claiming that GMO foods will enable us to feed more and more people. That may or may not be true, but what is certain is that studies and scientists have suggested GMOs have negative effects on our organ-functions. There's no benefit to feeding more people if the health of those people is compromised in the process.

Our brains seem to have reached oversaturation from so much technology and a sort of "brain freeze" from the pollutants that go along with "progress."

For those of us who are particularly sensitive to the environment, foods, and chemicals, it can be extremely challenging to feel good and be healthy. Many people with autoimmune disorders flee to a more agrarian way of life, away from the big cities, looking for places that are more conducive to a healthier lifestyle.

The *good news* is, of course, that there are positive steps we can take to have a cleaner environment. A primary example is to use more eco-friendly products around your home. Water and vinegar are an excellent combination, with no harmful chemicals, for cleaning floors and some surfaces. Whole Foods Market, many regular supermarkets, and other health-centered stores carry nontoxic cleaning products. Particularly if you have young children, read labels and be more conscientious about what you buy. Later in this chapter is a list of harmful chemicals to avoid whenever possible. Following is a list of toxins found in cleaning products.

ENVIRONMENTAL AND PRODUCT HAZARDS:

Below is a list of some harmful chemicals often found in cleaning or other products. In this section, you'll learn about toxins in cosmetics, cleaning products, pet foods, and other items you use daily.

Your children's health is affected in the home. If your child has allergies, asthma, other respiratory problems or digestion issues, it's a good idea to do a home-check to see what might be contributing to illness or lowered immunity.

PRODUCT: Air freshener

INGREDIENTS: Formaldehyde (embalming fluid), phthalates

POTENTIAL HAZARDS: Irritant to eyes, nose, throat, and skin; might cause nausea, headaches, nosebleeds, dizziness, memory loss and respiratory problems; can disrupt hormones and reproduction

PRODUCT: Ammonia

INGREDIENTS: Phenols

POSSIBLE HAZARDS: Irritating to eyes, skin, nose, respiratory tract, and throat; flammable and toxic

PRODUCT: Antifreeze

INGREDIENTS: Ethylene glycol

POTENTIAL HAZARDS: Contains lead, cadmium, and chromium in toxic levels; might be harmful to cardiovascular system, blood, skin, and kidneys

PRODUCT: Bleach, disinfectant

INGREDIENTS: Sodium hypochlorite

POSSIBLE HAZARDS: Might cause skin irritation or burns, damage to respiratory tract, pulmonary edema, vomiting, and gastrointestinal problems; contact with other chemicals can result in toxic chlorine fumes

PRODUCT: Car wax, polish

INGREDIENTS: Petroleum distillates

POTENTIAL HAZARDS: Might cause headaches, dizziness, nausea, irritated throat, and liver and kidney damage

PRODUCT: Drain cleaner

INGREDIENTS: Hydroxide (lye), hydrochloric acid, trichloromethane

POSSIBLE HAZARDS: Might slow reflexes or burn skin; poisonous if swallowed; might cause severe damage to liver, kidneys, digestive tract, and central nervous system

PRODUCT: Flea powder

INGREDIENTS: Carbaryl, dichlorophen, chlordane

POSSIBLE HAZARDS: Toxic insecticide; might impair nervous system; can cause headaches, memory loss, or muscle weakness; might damage skin, respiratory tract, kidney, liver, or spleen

PRODUCT: Floor cleaner or wax

INGREDIENTS: Diethylene glycol, petroleum solvents, ammonia

POSSIBLE HAZARDS: Toxic; might cause liver damage, central nervous system weakness, skin cancer, or lung cancer; irritant to eyes, nose, and respiratory tract

PRODUCT: Furniture polish

INGREDIENTS: Petroleum distillates

POSSIBLE HAZARDS: Highly flammable; irritant to nose, eyes, throat; and lungs; might cause skin and lung cancer

PRODUCT: Methanol

INGREDIENTS: Methyl hydroxide

POTENTIAL HAZARDS: Can cause headaches and dizziness; might damage liver, respiratory system, and central nervous system

PRODUCT: Motor oil, gasoline

INGREDIENTS: Benzene, lead

POSSIBLE HAZARDS: Highly flammable; might cause skin and lung cancer; irritant to nose, eyes, and skin; damaging to brain and nervous system

PRODUCT: Oven cleaner

INGREDIENTS: Poisonous hydroxide (lye)

POSSIBLE HAZARDS: Might cause severe lung, heart, or digestive damage; linked to blood in stools, esophageal burns, and swelling of the throat

PRODUCT: Paint

INGREDIENTS: Aromatic hydrocarbon thinners, mineral spirits, benzene

POSSIBLE HAZARDS: Might cause liver, lung, throat, and kidney damage; irritant to skin and eyes

PRODUCT: Paint thinner

INGREDIENTS: Chlorinated aliphatic hydrocarbons, alcohols, ketones, esters

POSSIBLE HAZARDS: Might cause damage to throat, eyes, nose, liver, kidney, lungs, or respiratory systems; carcinogenic

PRODUCT: Spot remover

INGREDIENTS: Perchlorethylene, trichloromethane, ammonium hydroxide, sodium hypochlorite

POSSIBLE HAZARDS: Might cause liver, kidney, or heart damage; irritating to skin, eyes, and lungs

PRODUCT: Toilet bowl cleaner

INGREDIENTS: Sodium acid sulfate, oxalate or hypochloric acid, chlorinated phenols.

POSSIBLE HAZARDS: May harm skin, lungs, circulation and heart; highly flammable.

PRODUCT: Window cleaner

INGREDIENTS: Diethylene glycol, ammonia

POSSIBLE HAZARDS: Irritating to eyes, nose, and respiratory tract; might harm liver and kidneys; burns skin

PRODUCT: Wood stain, varnish

INGREDIENTS: Mineral spirits, gasoline, benzene, lead

POSSIBLE HAZARDS: Highly flammable; might cause skin or lung cancer; can cause swelling in throat; stays in fatty tissue, bone marrow, and liver; damages digestive, neuromuscular, and central nervous systems

---

This book is a "call to action." If every person who connects with this information takes action in his or her own life, it will create a ripple that makes a wave, which builds up to a tsunami of change for all.

TOXINS IN FOOD PRODUCTS:

Acesulfame K: Alternative to sugar found in instant coffee mixes, nondairy creamers, pudding, gum, gelatin, and certain tea mixes

Acrylamide/polyacrylamide: High temperatures when cooking certain foods create this substance; also in some industrial products such as paper and dyes; found in inorganic coffee, potatoes, and dried fruit

Aluminum: Found in the environment from industry and in some processed foods, pickles, cheese, and baking soda; might contribute to Alzheimer's or other neurological damage

Aspartame: GMO substance and artificial sweetener, found in sodas, chewing gum; known to alter brain function, cause dizziness, destroy gut flora, affect blood sugar, and may be related to seizures, headaches, and cancer

BHT or Butylated Hydroxytoluene Technical Grade and BHA or Butylated Hydroxyanisole: Carcinogenic preservatives added to some foods; toxic to organs and skin; found in butter, processed meats, potato chips, beer, and petroleum products

Diacetyl: Artificial flavoring found in some foods, especially microwave popcorn, as well as candies, pet foods, and baked goods; might contribute to lung cancer, asthma, or other respiratory conditions

Fluoride: Might contain lead, mercury, cadmium, and arsenic; added to toothpastes and drinking water; might contribute to neurological disorders, kidney disease, cancer, bone loss, or cell degeneration

GMO (genetically modified organisms): Negatively manipulate gene and organ function; might contribute to cancer, brain disorders, and birth defects

High fructose corn syrup: Found in many foods, particularly sweets; might contribute to heart disease, raises cholesterol and triglycerides, causes blood clotting, feeds cancer cells, and harms gut flora

Hydrogenated or partially hydrogenated oils: Contain toxic trans fats; might relate to cancer, multiple sclerosis, neurological disorders, respiratory problems, high cholesterol, or heart disease

Magnesium stearate/stearic acid: Found in food and nutritional supplements; might have immune-suppressant effect on T-cells, which balance the immune system

Nitrates: Found in some medications, known to contribute to stomach cancer, dizziness, headaches, low blood pressure, and nausea

Olestra: Fat substitute; can contribute to abdominal pain, cramping, and weight gain; affects food absorption

PEG-80 Sorbitan Laurate: Added to some cosmetics, shampoos, and soaps as a fragrance and cleansing agent; might relate to allergies and immune deficiencies

Perchlorate: By-product of jet fuel found in lettuce, milk products, eggs, water, and air; affects thyroid function, hormones, respiratory tract, gastrointestinal tract, eyes, skin, and throat.

PFOA (perfluorooctanoic acid): By-product of processing Teflon; found in some foods and drinking water; stays in body and air for long periods of time; might contribute to cancer

Potassium bromate: Additive in bread; might contribute to cancer and affect immunity

Sodium nitrate: Found in processed meats, like bacon and jerky; damages blood vessels, blood sugar, heart, and arteries

Soy: Often genetically modified and might contain harmful herbicides (fermented soy is recommended); might relate to brain damage and breast cancer, calcium and vitamin D loss, thyroid deficiencies, infertility, and allergies

Sulfites: Preservatives used in foods and medications; might contribute to allergies, asthma, anaphylaxis, hives, and skin irritations

CHAPTER 2

CANDIDA: THE SILENT ENEMY

"Candida" (short for candidiasis) is a disorder caused by an overgrowth of yeast, candida albicans, in the body. Candida can live in the mouth, skin, genital area, gastrointestinal tract, brain, and can affect every organ in the body.

An average amount of candida in the body is harmless, but when an excess of candida accumulates, it secretes mycotoxins into the bloodstream, damaging the immune system and eventually leading to diseases. A mycotoxin is a secondary toxin produced from fungus, sometimes mold or other fungi. One mold species may produce many different mycotoxins, which, in turn, may be produced by several species of mold or fungi. Some mycotoxins are harmful to other fungi or bacteria. They resist being broken down by digestion, so they remain in the food chain in dairy and meat. Often cooking or freezing foods doesn't destroy some mycotoxins.

The environment is another source of mycotoxins, such as in buildings, homes or other living spaces. They are often difficult to identify, and therefore, eliminate. Mycotoxins disturb cell interactions, as well as RNA/DNA synthesis, and contribute to a host of domino-like effects in the body.

The majority of candida begins in the gut, which is at least 80 percent of our immune system. If the stomach has an overabundance of yeast fungus, it becomes porous, leaks through the gut wall, and the toxins flow through the bloodstream to any organ or part of the body, including the brain (Dr. David Perlmutter, a prominent, renowned neurologist, talks about the gut/brain connection in his book, Brain Maker). This phenomenon is called "leaky gut syndrome."

As the candida fungus continues to multiply and spread throughout the body, the immune system continues a gradual decline and becomes susceptible to a host of illnesses and disorders. The nature and scope of candida is extremely complex and often undetectable until it has caused irreparable damage.

If you've seen a medical doctor or more than one, and you tell him that you have candida and he tells you there is no such thing or that that's not your problem, see someone else (I've witnessed this many, many times from my own clients). If you know your body, are familiar with the symptoms and are sure you have fungus, find a practitioner who understands and can address the problem.

Many Western medical doctors are not familiar with candida or simply don't believe it exists. If left untreated, candida commonly leads to autoimmune disorders. Western doctors might treat the symptoms of an autoimmune disorder, but are not equipped to deal with the root or underlying cause of the illness (often candida). It's not part of their training in medical school (unless they're trained in integrative, functional medicine, which does deal with core issues).

When we look at the core or root causes of various diseases, including cancer, they always begin with a compromised immune system as a result of fungus, mold, bacteria, inflammation, parasites, or virus. Candida is, more often than not, the first pathogen in line.

Why is candida the primary cause of most illnesses? Candida is as insidious as a worm in an apple because it burrows deep into all areas of the body and multiplies rapidly. It feeds off of many of the forbidden foods we love to eat. It also comes from antibiotic overload as well as too much sugar, processed foods, sodas, cakes, cookies and dairy, and generally, poor nutrition.

In a country where fast food is the rule, not the exception, and antibiotics are prescribed every time a person sneezes, it's no wonder we are plagued by an increase of cancer and other autoimmune diseases.

What are the numerous causes of this condition? Oral antibiotics are probably the biggest culprits, because they kill off much of the good bacteria in the intestines, along with the bad. When bacteria are destroyed by antibiotics, the yeast remains and has more room to grow and feed off the foods in your body. This creates a vicious cycle as the yeast multiplies and manifests itself in various conditions. The symptoms of candida overgrowth can resemble a virus, bacteria, or other pathogens and, unfortunately, some doctors will prescribe antibiotics. Antibiotics only address bacteria, not viral or fungal conditions, and kill off good bacteria in the gut and intestines and again, give candida the opportunity to proliferate.

Pregnancy and menopause make it easier for the yeast to spread because they create an environment in which estrogen levels vary from the norm and impact the vaginal environment, resulting in higher rates of infection.

Immunity and candida are directly related, and if the balance in the body is compromised in any way, the immune system is at risk and the stage is set for candida to multiply. The health and strength of the immune system are contingent on balance in the entire body, particularly the gut, which is the seat of most illness.

If candida is overgrown, the immune system suffers, and the reverse is also applicable. If the immune system is weak, candida has the opportunity to increase at a greater rate than normal.

Other contributors to candida are steroids (cortisone and prednisone), birth control pills, chemotherapy, radiation, heavy metals, and the overuse of alcohol and drugs. Stress of any kind also causes candida to multiply because of its impact on the organs, hormones and endocrine system.

A host of environmental toxins, such as pesticides, herbicides, dioxins, and carbons, negatively affect the immune system and also invite the opportunity for yeast to multiply.

The candida creates toxins that pass through the liver, which has the burden of filtering all of the body's toxins. If the function of the liver is impaired due to toxic overload or poor nutrition, toxins can settle in the brain, nervous system, joints, skin, or other organs. The result, of course, might be chronic and debilitating disease.

More specifically, candida overgrowth targets the nerves and muscles—it's notorious for contributing to multiple sclerosis and other neurological disorders—and, again, might attack any organ in the body.

With multiple sclerosis, candida accumulates in the central nervous system, where it creates lesions in the myelin sheath. The myelin sheath insulates the nerves in the brain and spinal cord. These lesions grow and deepen, causing damage to the nerves and spinal cord, and begin the gradual process of disease.

Dr. David Perlmutter has done a great deal of research on the effects of candida on the brain. He states that patients with irritable bowel syndrome, or IBS, have fungus lesions almost as often as patients with multiple sclerosis (MS). Perlmutter maintains that this evidence provides a direct relationship between abnormalities in the gut and neurological disease.

Dr. Perlmutter's research reveals an important relationship between MS and problems in the digestive system, such as IBS, Crohn's disease, yeast overgrowth, and low levels of healthy bacteria. When levels of healthy flora in the gut and intestines are low, the gut is more susceptible to disease. Perlmutter states that candida has been associated with immune diseases, specifically MS, because of its impact on deterioration in the brain.

The *good news* is that there have been numerous documented cases where a person suffering from severe MS has completely reversed the condition with detoxification, proper nutrition, herbs, supplements, acupuncture and acupressure, along with emotional and spiritual guidance.

SIGNS AND SYMPTOMS OF CANDIDA:

The signs, symptoms, and effects of severe candida are numerous, insidious, far-reaching, and severely debilitating. Many health issues, both serious and mild, masquerade as rashes, colds, breathing problems, hives, viral or bacterial infections, autoimmune disorders, and more. Doctors sometimes treat them as such, too often prescribing antibiotics, ointments, inhalers, or other medications. This usually addresses an immediate discomfort, but not the core issue, which can originate with an overgrowth of candida.

In the long run, these measures have only a palliative effect without addressing the underlying pathogen. The treatment is to starve the fungus with an altered diet, administer antifungal supplements or medication, and detoxify the gut and body.

It's a daunting state of affairs that many Western medical doctors with good intentions are taught to treat only the problem but not to find the solution. Medical schools, for the most part, focus on diagnosis and palliative medicine (which helps a patient be comfortable) but not on nutrition, supplements, and alternative treatments such as herbs and uncommon therapies.

There is hope, however, because integrative, functional medical practices are increasing as the need for them becomes more prevalent. *Some medical schools across the country now have an entire department dedicated to integrative, functional medicine.* This is wonderful and revolutionary news.

As more and more people have become sicker and more severely debilitated by autoimmune diseases, greater numbers of Western medical doctors have studied both Western and alternative medicine of all kinds, and have adopted a holistic approach to treating illness.

There is a great deal of evidence that many of these alternative therapies, which are discussed later in the book, are very often effective, curative, and when maintained, offer long-lasting benefits.

SYMPTOMS OF YEAST OVERGROWTH:
Additional symptoms of yeast overgrowth can include:

- low energy
- fatigue
- anxiety
- irritability
- fear

- depression
- headaches
- lightheadedness
- muscle and joint pain (arthritis)
- chemical sensitivity
- poor circulation resulting in consistently cold hands and feet
- urinary tract infections
- rectal itching
- white coating on the tongue or esophagus
- heart palpitations
- irregular heartbeat

OTHER SIGNS AND SYMPTOMS OF CANDIDA OVERGROWTH ARE:

- mental and emotional imbalances
- anxiety
- depression
- brain fog
- forgetfulness
- confusion
- irritability
- irrational thinking

Because mycotoxins are capable of crossing the blood-brain barrier, candida can cause chemical imbalances in the brain, neurological diseases, and a slow process of physical and mental decline.

In the digestive tract, symptoms include:

- gas
- bloating
- constipation or diarrhea

- nausea, loss of appetite, indigestion
- intestinal cramps

In the respiratory tract, symptoms include:

- chronic postnasal drip
- coughs
- sore throats
- colds
- pneumonia
- difficulty breathing
- allergies
- asthma
- appearance of scarring on the lungs

On the skin, symptoms include:

- eczema
- psoriasis
- dry
- flaky patches
- itching
- rashes
- acne
- discoloration
- fungal infections

A variety of gynecological problems might occur in both men and women, the most common of which is chronic yeast infection. This causes redness, itching, irritation, and discharge in the vaginal area or penis. It's important to note that candida is easily transmitted from one partner to another, so caution is encouraged. Although products on the market can eliminate immediate symptoms, they will not address the underlying cause of the fungus, which begins in the gut and works its way outward.

Heavy metals in the body (from food, chemicals, and environmental exposure) are also related to overgrowth of candida toxins. These elements inhibit proper function of the immune system and create an opportunity for the fungus to invade and propagate.

PARTIAL LIST OF TOXIC HEAVY METALS:

- Aluminum
- Antimony
- Arsenic
- Barium
- Beryllium
- Cadmium
- Hexavalent chromium
- Lead
- Mercury
- Strontium

VACCINATIONS:
The reason for the current controversy over the use of vaccinations is that we don't know exactly what comprises these vaccines, but we do know that there are some toxic chemical components. There have not been enough broad-spectrum studies conducted on the effects of vaccinations on children. We do know that numerous reports have come from mothers who were convinced their children became very sick, or in some cases even died, as a result of vaccinations. Vaccinations are relevant because they have, in many cases, reportedly broken down the immune system, which is an opportune time for the overgrowth of candida, even in little children.

MERCURY TOXICITY AFFECTS CANDIDA OVERGROWTH:

An overwhelming amount of heavy metals in the body can cause candida overgrowth, due to weakening immunity. Many studies have reported the effects of mercury on the brain. It's estimated to be one of the most toxic and damaging substances known to humans. These studies find that mercury might contribute to autism and Asperger syndrome in children, as well MS, Alzheimer's, and numerous other autoimmune and neurological disorders. The candida, which is the primary or secondary infection, simultaneously wreaks havoc on the entire body.

Many mental health care professionals will ascribe a mental illness to specific symptoms, behaviors, and textbook pathologies without acknowledging that aberrant thoughts and behaviors might be attributed to toxic overload, rather than clinical pathology.

Some studies report specific cases of complete recovery after a physical detoxification process. Because the body and mind are intertwined and connected, the body often dictates how the mind operates and functions. If toxins, candida, viruses, and bacteria create physical pathology, it stands to reason that the mind is also affected. We know we can heal the body with detoxification, proper nutrition, herbs, and supplements, and can apply the same treatments to our mental functions.

Holistic practitioners have the knowledge to understand how the mind affects physical health, and are able to encourage healing without the use of pharmaceutical drugs.

The purpose of this information is to support you in your healing process. Education, knowledge, and awareness are the keys to getting the appropriate help you need. Comprehensive and sustained health is highly possible when you know how to achieve it. If you, your family, or friends have issues that are untreated or unresolved, or if you feel you're in the wrong hands, it's important to do the research to take the next indicated action.

TREATMENTS AND PROTOCOLS:

Now that you're informed about the problems created by candida, it's crucial that you understand how to turn to solutions. These protocols, diets, and supplements are practical, logical, and varied, and produce positive, immune-supportive results.

There are blood tests, hair and urine analyses, muscle tests, and bio-energy machines to help diagnose candida. Once you know a diagnosis is positive, you're ready to begin the process of healing.

The goal of treating yeast overgrowth is to kill off the excess in order to bring the body back into balance. These strategies are effective, thorough, safe, and recommended by alternative, integrative, and holistic practitioners.

Naturally, detoxification, which is addressed in more detail in the following chapter, is the first process on the list. Think of your body as you do your car: if you want to maintain a clean engine, you need to clean your oil periodically. If you want to clean your gut, you need to take action that eliminates toxins. This seems like a tall order for some, but it's not as difficult as you might think. Many products, foods, and supplements eliminate all kinds of toxins, and some form of detoxification is absolutely necessary to maintain a healthy body.

Many antifungal products are on the market. The most effective pharmaceutical product is Nystatin. Nystatin, which is a plant-based, natural substance and non-harmful, kills the fungus effectively and may be taken in pill form for as long as necessary (no more than two years).

HIGHLY RECOMMENDED NATURAL ANTIFUNGAL PRODUCTS:

- Twinlab **Yeast Fighters**
- Rainbow Light **Candida Cleanse**
- Garden of Life **Primal Defense**
- **Pau d'Arco** (herbal tea or capsule)
- Protocol for Life Balance **Candida Away**
- Pure Essence Labs **Candex**
- Enzymedica **Candidase**

NATURAL HERBS AND SUPPLEMENTS:

A few examples of some beneficial natural substances are garlic, Oregon grape root, berberine, grapefruit seed extract, caprylic acid, fennel, ginger, oregano oil, peppermint oil, coconut oil, chlorella, olive leaf extract, apple cider vinegar, marshmallow, gentian root, black walnut, citrus seed extract, black seed, and colloidal silver.

These remedies may be used in combination with one another, but use two or three at a time and rotate them. It isn't necessary to use all of them, and be sure to note how your body feels after ingesting any of them. They are more cost-effective than medicinal drugs, are nonprescription, and can be found in health food stores and online.

Always consult with a health care professional before administering these protocols on your own.

It's necessary to maintain a healthful diet, without sugar, gluten, sodas, dairy, soy, trans fats, coffee, processed foods and fried foods, while you're detoxifying. Keep your nutrition as clean and simple as possible. Eat lean meats (unless you're vegan or vegetarian), vegetables, and simple grains like quinoa, amaranth, spelt, millet, and buckwheat. Be careful of fruits because they contain sugar, and even natural sugars can increase candida overgrowth.

The "die-off" reactions of detoxification are worth noting. The process of detoxifying might make you feel worse before you feel better. You might possibly experience flu-like symptoms, body aches, headaches, stomach problems, and other discomfort. This is a normal reaction to die-off. Make sure you drink at least eight glasses of water daily to flush the toxins out of your body. Even if your bowels work normally, it's still recommended that you take one or two of the following for more thorough elimination:

Pau d'Arco tea is a good elimination tool, as are natural fiber, psyllium, senna, licorice, magnesium, warm lemon water, pure olive oil, flaxseed, aloe, dandelion, rhubarb, red clover tea, and caffeine-free green tea.

These are only some of the products that help the digestive and intestinal tracts eliminate toxins. It's essential to do this extra cleansing regime because you want the toxins removed, not floating around in your body.

If you notice the die-off symptoms are too intense and uncomfortable, stop taking the remedies for a few days, but stay with the diet and flush your body with plenty of water, only.

Another channel of cleansing is through the lungs, which constitute 75 percent of the toxins you eliminate—make sure you sit in a comfortable position where it's quiet and dimly lighted, then take several deep breaths. Take the air in from your nose, and release it from your mouth. Repeat this breathing exercise 3 or 4 times, at least 3 times a day.

While you're in a relaxed state of mind, visualize your favorite scene-- a day at the beach with dolphins swimming before you and the sound of seagulls; hiking in the mountains surrounded by lots of greenery and fanciful birds singing; a rainbow spreading its beauty over a mystical sky. Visualize whatever scenario makes you light up, and feel peaceful and serene.

Engaging in this kind of yoga breathing and visualization provides an excellent way to focus on feeling calm. If you can practice breathing 3 times daily, your immune system will experience greater rejuvenation and regeneration.

Restful sleep is always important to healing and staying healthy. Get plenty of exercise, at least three times a week to sweat out the toxins, and clear the lymphatic system by getting a massage or brushing your body (several body brushes on the market) in the shower.

Acupuncture and acupressure are also highly recommended, as they aid the body in detoxification and healing. Cardio workouts increase your heartrate and strengthen your core, while pilates offers resistance training and comprehensive stretching. If you're a runner, run 3 times a week for strength and endurance. If you like to walk, walk twice a day for 30 minutes, which helps stimulate circulation and detoxification. The amount of time you spend on these exercises depends on the shape you're in, so if you're not used to it, start off with 15 minutes, then 30 minutes and finally, an hour.

Massage is important because it stimulates the lymphatic and circulatory systems which help eliminates toxins, while brushing your body in the shower relates to your largest organ—the skin. Brushing away dead skin is a healthy daily practice.

Now we come to the most significant part of the regimen: nutrition. The list of *do's* and *do not's* are somewhat repetitious, but nutrition is an important issue.

You might feel as if you can't eat anything you like, but if you like junk foods, dairy, sodas, bread, cakes, and everything that feeds inflammation and candida, you're taxing your immune system, over time. Once you become accustomed to "good" nutrition, you may no longer enjoy toxic foods which have no intrinsic value.

You don't have to remove all of the following foods from your diet forever, but while you're eliminating the fungus, it's important to be diligent about what you eat. While you're detoxifying, avoid these foods. You can introduce them back into your diet later. However, if you have known food allergies or sensitivities, avoid all foods that don't agree with you.

NIGHTSHADES CAN CAUSE LEAKY GUT SYNDROME:
Nightshades are foods like eggplant, tomatoes, goji berries, and other foods that contribute to inflammation in the body. Nightshades contain compounds that might contribute to pain, digestive issues, and inflammation. Since leaky gut is caused from an overgrowth of candida, it's relevant to note the nutritional values here, again.

The nightshade family is called "solanacea," and has more than two thousand species, many of which are inedible and highly poisonous. However, many edible plants are also part the nightshade family:

- Goji Berry
- Naranjilla
- Pimiento
- Tamarillo
- Tomatillo

COMPONENTS THAT MAKE NIGHTSHADES DIFFICULT TO DIGEST:

SOLANINE is a nerve toxin. Potatoes are nightshades that contain varying amounts of solanine and capsaicin (see below). The more green the potato, the more toxins it contains.

SAPONINS are compounds like pesticides and herbicides, designed to protect plants from microbes and insects. When consumed by humans, saponins can create holes in the gut wall, increasing leaky gut and allowing pathogens and toxins into the bloodstream. They can also cause inflammation in the body. Peppers are high in saponins. Ripe tomatoes have low levels of saponins, while green tomatoes and hothouse tomatoes (those harvested before they are ripe) are very high in saponins.

LECTINS, found in nightshades (also in beans), are a concern because they are difficult to digest. They're able to withstand the heat of cooking, which means they are intact when you eat them, and contribute to leaky gut. They can penetrate the protective mucus of the small intestine, where they promote cell division inappropriately and might cause cell death. Lectins can perforate the intestinal wall and trick the immune system into thinking there's an invader, potentially causing an allergic reaction.

CAPSAICIN is a stimulant that gives chili peppers their heat. It's a potent irritant to mucous membranes and can also contribute to leaky gut. While potatoes have some of these compounds and might lead to candida, yams and sweet potatoes are in a different family—those do, however, contain amounts of natural sugar and therefore, must be eaten in moderation.

FOODS TO AVOID:

Dairy, according to the majority of respected holistic doctors and practitioners, including Dr. David Perlmutter, is not good for much of anything, so avoid cheeses, buttermilk, cow's milk, ice cream, margarine, cream cheese, sour cream, and regular yogurt.

The most important **condiments** to avoid are catsup, mayonnaise, mustard, pickles, relish, vinegar and soy sauce. Apple cider vinegar is acceptable because of its alkalizing and anti-inflammatory properties.

Oils to avoid are corn, soy, peanut, canola (GMO-sourced), cottonseed, hydrogenated, and trans fat oils of any kind.

Nuts and **seeds** to avoid in particular are peanuts, pistachios, and cashews.

In the **grain** category, avoid pasta, breads, corn, cereals, crackers, pastries, white flour, white rice, gluten, and whole wheat.

Of course, what might be considered **junk food**, such as candy, coffee, fast food, fried food, chocolate, donuts, muffins, pizza, cakes, and cookies are off limits.

As for **beverages**, alcohol turns to sugar in the body and should be avoided; fruit juices and sodas contain large amounts of sugar.

Fruits that multiply candida are bananas, apricots, papaya, grapes, guava, berries, cherries, melons, mangos, peaches, pears, and plums. Eat an apple once or twice a week if you crave sugar, or eat protein instead, which might satisfy the craving.

If you must have any of these foods while you're on this cleanse, eat only one of them on any given day. Be mindful, discriminating and consistent.

- Canned tuna
- Shellfish
- Processed meat
- Bacon
- Hot dogs
- Sausage
- Mushrooms
- Corn
- Tomato
- Eggplant
- Potato

PARTIAL LIST OF FOODS YOU CAN AND SHOULD EAT ON CLEANSE:

Eat **poultry and other proteins** such as chicken, duck, lamb, eggs, turkey, and beef—grass-fed and hormone-free—unless you're vegan or vegetarian.

Most **leafy green vegetables** are good: spinach, kale, broccoli, green beans, chard, Brussels sprouts, asparagus, celery. Avoid an excess of sweet potatoes and yams, as they contain sugar.

Non-hydrogenated oils that are fine include organic coconut, olive, sesame, grape-seed, flax, red palm, and sunflower.

Whole grains recommended are spelt, rye, barley, kamut, brown rice, buckwheat, millet, quinoa, and amaranth.

Nuts and seeds include almond, Brazil, chestnut, macadamia, hazelnut, pecan, walnut, pumpkin seed, sesame seed, and sunflower seed.

Recommended condiments are apple cider vinegar, dry mustard, pepper, rice vinegar, sea salt, and fresh herbs.

Stevia and xylitol, in moderation, are preferable **sweeteners**.

Take probiotics daily. They should contain various strains of healthy bacteria, such as acidophilus, B. longum, L. fermentum, L. salivarius, L. plantarum, L. rhamnosus, and B. bifidum, which help restore natural flora back into the gut and intestines.

What will you experience when you go on a candida diet?

LIST OF POSSIBLE "DIE-OFF" SYMPTOMS:

- Headache
- Fatigue
- Nausea
- Dizziness
- Bloating
- Gas
- Constipation
- Diarrhea

- Chills
- Fever
- Sweating
- Muscle pain
- Eczema
- Psoriasis
- Sinus infections
- Vaginal infections
- Heart palpitations

These symptoms might not affect you, or you could experience some but not all of them. Once you conquer the detoxification process and feel better, the quality of your life will improve.

Because candida can cause so many health problems, the breadth and depth of the damage is not always obvious; once it's eliminated, your body will be on a healthy trajectory and you'll begin to notice how good you feel.

After the detoxification process, especially if you've had mild or serious illnesses, your body will be more sensitive to what you put into it. You won't be able to resume bad eating habits and stay healthy—but the chances are, you won't want to!

CHAPTER 3

DETOXIFICATION

Detoxification is a primary issue because it addresses the whole body and is the first step towards good health. Since toxins, bad bacteria, virus, chemicals, and parasites debilitate the body over a period of time, it's critical to cleanse before any treatment can be effective.

If your immune system is compromised by illness, it's especially important to begin with a candida cleanse and progress onto a complete body detoxification. If you're seriously ill, detoxification must be a gradual process, at your doctor's recommendation. All cleanses are similar but not quite the same. The remedies for a complete detoxification are a bit different from a candida cleanse because you're eliminating a broader spectrum of toxins.

Always consult with a health care practitioner, preferably someone who focuses on a holistic approach, before embarking on a cleansing protocol, particularly if you're immune-deficient and have health issues.

The liver is especially significant because it filters out toxins and helps them pass through the stomach and intestines. It's involved with digestion, immunity, metabolism, storing fats, cholesterol and protein (the liver breaks down protein and fats), bile production, breaking down insulin, converting sugar to balance blood sugar levels, destroying old blood cells, blood detoxification and purification, and storage of nutrients. The liver also metabolizes and circulates hormones throughout the body, helping them maintain a healthy balance.

Blood travels to the stomach, spleen, gallbladder, intestines, and pancreas through capillaries, collecting in the portal vein of the liver. The blood is then processed in the liver, where waste is separated from nutrients, and passes on to the rest of the body. The liver stores vitamins and minerals in order to supply these supplements to body tissues.

Kupffer cells, formed in the spleen and lymph nodes, help digest bacteria, fungi, parasites, and cellular waste. These cells clean the blood in the liver very quickly.

Because the liver works harder than any other organ to maintain balance, it's the most vulnerable organ in the body. It's also the most regenerative organ with the ability to grow and repair quickly. The liver has a dynamic effect on the immune system and is a crucial aspect of detoxification. All other organs are dependent on liver health to function properly.

SUPER-NUTRIENTS FOR CLEANING THE LIVER:

All of these foods contain nutrients that help clean the liver: carrot, beet, ripe tomato (in moderation, contain large amounts of glutathione which eliminates toxins and heavy metals from the liver), grapefruit, spinach, lemon, lime, cabbage, walnut, avocado, Brussels sprouts, apple, turmeric, cumin, coriander, cardamom, cayenne, cinnamon, fennel, garlic, ginger, leafy green vegetables,

cruciferous vegetables such as cauliflower and broccoli, asparagus, artichokes, parsley, dandelion, milk thistle, green tea, olive
oil, brown algae, sprouted nuts, beans, seeds, onion, and super-
charged probiotic and prebiotic supplements.

If you're on a treatment plan, these are all healthful, safe,
and nourishing choices. Don't try to eat all of these in one
day! Rotate your foods, and be mindful of how you feel along
the way.

PARTIAL LIST OF PRODUCTS THAT CLEAN THE LIVER:

In addition to the nutrient-rich foods listed above, there are
numerous products on the market, outlined below, that aid in liver
detoxification. Some are in pill form with explicit directions, and
some are powder. Your practitioner can give you directions on how
to take these supplements.

Ortho Molecular Products **PhytoCore**
Standard Process **SP Cleanse 150 C**
Dr. Schulze's **5-Day Liver Detox** (liver-gallbladder detox formula)
Thorne Research **Liver Cleanse**
Enzymatic Therapy **Complete Liver Cleanse**
Natawill Nutrition **Livergenex**
NOW Foods **Liver Detoxifier & Regenerator**
Planetary Formulas **Bupleurum Liver Cleanse**
Metagenics **Silymarin**
Gaia Herbs **Liver Health**
Pure Formulas **Herbal Hepaclenz**
Carlson **Norwegian Cod Liver Oil**
NutriCology **Magnesium Chloride**

These products may be taken alongside the recommended diet. Your doctor can help you choose which one is the best remedy for you. Sometimes it's a process of trial and error, because we all respond differently to different substances.

As an additional benefit, the gallbladder and liver work together, so you're cleansing both at the same time.

Cleaning the gut and intestines is vital, and the large intestine affects the lungs because of the absorption of fluids in the body. In Chinese medicine, their energies are paired. Cleaning the large intestine, therefore, helps supports lung function. Although a liver cleanse ultimately filters through the kidneys, gut and intestines, there are specific supplements and herbs for cleaning the kidneys. The diet is almost the same for all detoxification.

PARTIAL LIST OF FOODS FOR GUT AND COLON CLEANSE:

Some of these are repeated from the candida cleanse, but the following are specific to cleansing the gut and colon: fiber-rich food; full-spectrum probiotics; apple cider vinegar; apple, flaxseed, chia seed, chlorophyll, spirulina, blue-green algae; lemon water with sea salt, limited fermented food; sprouts, green tea; unsulfured dried fruit like cranberry; kelp, nori, adzuki bean, pumpkin seed, sunflower seed, hemp seed, tahini, hemp oil, almond oil, chia oil, avocado oil, and coconut oil.

Most of the liver diet is also helpful for this gut/colon cleanse, with another cautionary note about strictly limiting or eliminating sugar (even in fruits); caffeine, gluten, processed food, nonorganic food, and dairy.

PRODUCTS FOR GUT AND COLON CLEANSE:

Blessed Herbs **Colon Cleansing Kit**
Enzymatic Therapy **Whole Body Cleanse**
Futurebiotics **Colon Green**
Ortho Molecular Products **Core Restore BT 7-Day Kit**
Dr. Schulze's **Intestinal Formula #1**
Organic India **Bowelcare**
Tibetan Herbal Balance **Colon Support**
Aerobic Life **Aerobic Bulk Cleanse**
Gaia Herbs **Daily Cleanse Fiber**

There are other formulas, both herbal and supplemental, to help with the gut and colon cleansing process, along with diet, exercise, plenty of water daily, and intentional healing. Your spiritual, emotional and mental practices contribute greatly to the state of your health, so if you're on a wellness mission, incorporate these into your daily life.

The kidneys are the next important organ, closely connected to the liver and affecting all other organs. The kidneys process the blood to help remove water and waste from food and tissues.

They also release hormones, which help maintain proper levels of calcium in the body. These hormones affect bone marrow (red blood cells), regulate blood pressure, and support vitamin D for bones and balance.

Again, the diet is almost the same, and there are specific supplemental herbs and formulas that might be helpful.

It's important to do these cleanses one at a time with a few weeks' time in between each—otherwise, you might go on toxic overload.

The length of time for detoxification depends upon your doctor's recommendation and the nature of your own process. Everyone is different and requires an individual treatment plan; there is no one-for-all protocol.

SPECIFIC FOODS TO CLEAN THE KIDNEYS:

The following are particularly good for kidney cleansing: nettle tea, dandelion tea; parsley, ginger, watermelon, red clover; black currant juice, cranberry juice; marshmallow root, turmeric, spirulina; blueberry, lemon, grape, asparagus, millet, barley, and pumpkin seed.

KIDNEY FORMULA PRODUCTS FOR CLEANSING:

Dr. Schulze's **5-Day Kidney Detox**
Metagenics **Renagen DTX**
Solaray **Kidney Blend SP-6**
Pure Formulas **Kidney Formula**
Enzymatic Therapy **Aqua-Flow**

There are natural ways in which to clean the kidneys—certain foods, liquids, and water are the best sources for cleaning the body, as long as they're natural, safe, effective, and support your immune system during the process. The supplements, formulas, herbs or other products may be added at your doctor's discretion.

PARASITE CLEANSE

The last important cleanse is for the elimination of parasites. These are living organisms that feed off of your body, most often at your expense. Parasites can live almost anywhere inside you, and are too often overlooked during medical diagnoses. They originate from many different sources, grow in all kinds of environments, and can pose extreme and extraordinary health problems.

EXAMPLES OF PARASITES:

Hookworms, pinworms, tapeworms, flukes, roundworms, whipworms, trichinella, filariasis, dog roundworms

These are only a few. They're insidious, often invisible to the eye, burrow deep into the body, multiply quickly, and feed off the host, creating toxic bacterial pathogens that may lead to serious disease. Parasites can destroy brain tissue, red and white blood cells, the gut and intestines, and eat away at your organs.

It's crucial to wash fruits and vegetables thoroughly, protect your skin with natural sprays or lotions, eat organic as much as possible, pay attention to fish and meat sources, and keep your kitchen clean.

SYMPTOMS OF PARASITES:

These are only a few possible symptoms: stomach pain, nausea, diarrhea, vomiting, dysentery (bloody stools), fatigue, rashes, weight loss, muscle pain, paralysis, headaches, and flu-like symptoms. Parasites are clever bugs because they adapt to changes in the body, in order to survive.

Because they have the ability to adapt to changes in the environment, parasites are often difficult to find and identify until symptoms become serious or life-threatening.

Parasites are known to mirror or mimic specific illnesses as they swim around in the bloodstream, wreaking havoc along the way.

They are easily misdiagnosed, and treated as something differ-ent from what they are, thus further causing inflammation and disease.

Parasites love sugar and everything that turns into sugar. The best way to starve parasites is healthy fasting and cleansing strategies, while eliminating sugar and grains from your diet.

HERBS AND FOODS WITH SIGNIFICANT ANTIPARASITIC AGENTS:

Extra virgin coconut oil is full of medium-chain triglycerides that strengthen the immune system in its battle against pathogens. Raw garlic and onions provide sulfur-containing amino acids that are anti-parasitic. It's recommended to eat six tablespoons of raw extra virgin coconut oil, one whole clove of garlic, and one large red onion daily to help parasite-proof your body. Eat these in foods, if you like; if you're sensitive to onions or garlic, reduce to half the amount. Dried oregano and especially essential oil of oregano are extremely anti-parasitic. Use two to three drops of oregano oil in water with fresh-squeezed lemon and drink it three times a day. Cloves are just as effective, and you can substitute, or use clove oil with oregano oil. Ginger, wormwood, and black walnut are also commonly used to treat parasites.

Fasting with fermented drinks such as fermented ginger, coconut kefir, and apple cider vinegar are also effective anti-parasitics. Kombucha is questionable because it contains high amounts of sugar, which feed parasites.

Many holistic practitioners recommend a three- to twenty-one-day low-calorie liquid diet rich in fermented beverages, water, and fresh squeezed lemon. Probiotic supplements are highly recommended to help destroy parasites and put healthy bacteria back into the gut.

If your immune system is compromised, fasting is a choice you and your doctor must consider carefully.

After the cleansing period, it's especially important to continue to utilize high-quality fermented foods and vegetables. Raw fermented products like amasai, kimchi, sauerkraut, and fermented veggies may be consumed. These foods are rich sources of L-glutamine, an amino acid that helps rebuild the gut. They also contain very powerful strains of good bacteria, organic acids, and enzymes that eliminate parasites.

There are parasite cleanses on the market that are highly effective, and it's best to consult your practitioner about the best one for you. Parasites, like candida, can be the root cause of a host of immune problems because they weaken and deplete the body of essential nutrients, and create inflammation.

PRODUCTS THAT HELP CLEAR PARASITES:

Renew Life **ParaGone**
Herbal Healer Academy **Intestinal Freedom**
Nutracraft **ParasiteClear**
ParaZyte **Detox Complex**
Dr. Clark Store **Original Parasite Cleanse**
OneLifeUSA **Parasite Cleanse Kit**
Mountain Song **PARA Response**
Natural Healthy Concepts **Paracid Forte**

These are only a few available products. If your symptoms are serious and persistent, and the source of your sickness hasn't been identified, ask your doctor to take a stool test and check your blood for parasites. Someone such as a gastrointestinal (GI) specialist will eventually get to the bottom of it and prescribe the proper medication or remedy.

If you're sick, have chronic illness, and are undiagnosed, it's recommended that you test for parasites, candida, and exposure to heavy metals and other chemicals that weigh heavily on the immune system.

HEAVY METAL DETOXIFICATION

Heavy metals are a completely different issue. We're exposed to them daily in the environment. They come from various sources of foods, water, air, and products of all kinds.

One of the best treatments for heavy metal toxicity is glutathione, a substance often called the "master builder" because it has so many natural medicinal properties. It attaches to the metals in the body and eliminates them. It's safe, effective, powerful, and available in foods and supplements.

LivOn Labs is a company that makes bioavailable products, which are easily metabolized and absorbed by the body. **Lypo-Spheric GSH** is a gel form of glutathione that you can put into juice or smoothies, and it's highly effective.

Chelation therapy is another form of heavy metal detoxification and will be discussed later on in the book.

There are several autoimmune disorders, particular neurological, that are the result of toxic metals, which cross the blood-brain barrier.

The good news is, of course, that autoimmune diseases are cured every day. In the following chapter, you'll read about the success stories of people who have cured themselves with the help of a professional support team, and daily attention to physical, mental, emotional and spiritual practices.

CHAPTER 4

PERSONAL TRIUMPHS OVER AUTOIMMUNE DISORDERS

These are true stories of people, who, except for one, have conquered serious and debilitating autoimmune disorders with the help of doctors, practitioners, friends, loved ones and through their own search for balance in their lives. Healing happens when the body/mind/spirit connection is aligned and working synergistically. This is what separates people who heal, from those who, sadly, aren't able to find the support and connection needed in order to achieve balance.

SUSAN

Susan suffered from a series of symptoms that seemed to baffle even the best doctors and specialists. She developed pain, stiffness, and rope-like twists in her hands and feet. Susan decided to take control of her situation and became her own advocate, when professionals had failed to find a solution. She, eventually, was compelled to do a great deal of research and talked with a variety of alternative health care professionals and practitioners.

At that time, fifteen years ago, a diagnosis of this particular issue was difficult because the symptoms were uncommon. Susan had experienced severe pain and discomfort in her hands while at work, becoming less and less able to perform her job. She was a hairstylist for celebrities in the film industry, so it was important for her to be able to use her hands.

After a year or so of feeling weak, debilitated, and undiagnosed, Susan knew it was time to get some answers. She also knew it was time to think about a new career. Finally, after a lot of unsuccessful searching, a rheumatologist in Beverly Hills, California, recommended by a friend, accurately diagnosed the problem.

The doctor told Susan she had a rather uncommon autoimmune disorder called Dupuytren's Contracture, and that the only solution he knew of was surgery. He told her that the procedure would necessitate cutting the tendons in her hands to give them flexibility, and that they would eventually heal so that her life would return to normal.

That wasn't the scenario Susan had in mind—invasive surgery and waiting for her hands to heal. The next step was to further investigate all of her options. Susan was more invested in natural herbs and supplements, and the idea of surgery was not a viable choice for her at that time.

In desperation, Susan contacted the brother-in-law of a close friend, a holistic medical doctor who recommended a few alternative medical doctors.

After meeting with different practitioners, Susan met an alternative medical doctor, who was able to not only make a diagnosis but also pinpoint the root cause of the disorder—and the solutions didn't require surgery.

The doctor told Susan that the core of Dupuytren's was caused from chemical toxins in the environment that settle on the skin and in the lungs, inserting themselves into the immune system.

Hairstylists work with many toxins: aluminum, permanent wave solution, bleach, dyes, hair sprays, relaxers, glue, and other chemicals.

Susan had been exposed to these chemicals regularly from a very young age, as her parents owned a hair salon on Long Island, New York, and she had spent much of her childhood working in that environment.

The practitioner's recommendation, and one of the only ways to detoxify all of the toxins from the fatty tissues in the body, was to sweat them out.

Susan was referred to a special facility, where the detoxification process was monitored; for five weeks, five hours a day, she ingested—building doses gradually—massive doses of niacin to flush the body, volumes of water, healthful snacks, and a specific combination of powerful antioxidant vitamins.

The protocol was designed for maximum efficiency with these steps: Susan was inside the sauna in increasing increments, but for not more than twenty minutes at a time. She ate and drank water in between, and spent a certain amount of time on a treadmill to continually increase the sweating, stimulate circulation, and eliminate the toxins.

This was a grueling, exhausting, time-consuming, and challenging process. During the weeks of cleansing, Susan said she could smell every chemical, every drug, and toxic substance she had ever taken in her life, and, literally, felt all of them pour out of her body while she sweated.

As the days passed into the third or fourth week, Susan's hands and feet began to open, and she felt relief for the first time in over a year. By the fifth week, her hands and feet were almost back to normal. There was only a very small amount of discomfort, but her hands and feet were opened and she could use them easily. By the end of the fifth week, Susan felt like herself again.

Susan had been a true warrior, and along with this process, she spent time in meditation and prayer daily, visualizing the chemicals pouring out of her body. She also received acupuncture treatments. Although there were days when she felt very sick and discouraged, Susan always believed she would heal, and that her body would become whole again. With the support of loved ones and friends and numerous emotional and spiritual healings, Susan had, after several months, achieved optimum health.

Although some might call it a miracle, and Western medical doctors might be surprised, skeptical, or in disbelief, the reality is that Susan addressed the core, or root, of her illness, and the results were clearly in evidence.

Her hands and feet have remained quite functional, and Susan is now a thriving real estate agent in Los Angeles. She had been forced to change her career in order to live a cleaner, healthier life, and this decision had saved her life.

Susan maintains her health by cleansing periodically, keeping her diet in balance, and by being conscious of her lifestyle. Today, she is grateful, attentive of self-care, and happily paying it forward into the next chapter of her life.

If you have a heart condition or other medical problems, you must always consult with your doctor before engaging in this kind of treatment.

ASHLEY

This is the story about a woman named Ashley, who led a healthy, normal life until age thirty-three. At that time, and quite unexpectedly, Ashley's life changed drastically.

Ashley and Carrie worked as physical therapists in the same clinic. They were good friends, worked hard, ate lunch together, and looked out for each other's welfare.

One day as Ashley and Carrie were on their way to lunch, Carrie noticed Ashley inadvertently bumping into her as they walked. Ashley's balance seemed to be off, and Carrie realized this had been going on for quite some time. She asked Ashley if she realized she was wobbling and if she had noticed any other symptoms.

Carrie had been studying Chinese herbs at the time, learning about nutrition and autoimmune disorders. She was aware of Ashley's diet, which had been unhealthful and imbalanced, and began to put the pieces together. It occurred to Carrie that Ashley needed to see a neurologist.

Ashley protested, convinced she was fine and that she intended to eat more healthfully and avoid cakes, cookies, and candy. Carrie wasn't convinced, but in the interest of keeping peace, she let it go.

As time passed, Ashley's balance became worse, her muscles got weaker, she was easily fatigued, her face was pale, and she looked anemic and gaunt.

Carrie talked with Ashley again, this time not accepting "no" for an answer. She insisted Ashley see a neurologist as soon as possible. Carrie was convinced Ashley had an autoimmune disorder that needed immediate attention.

After an exam by a neurologist and several tests later, Ashley was told she had multiple sclerosis and needed to be on a treatment program right away. There are a few different medical treatments for MS, one of which is interferon. It reduces inflammation in MS patients and has an antiviral action to minimize the effects of the virus. Interferon is also used to treat certain cancers, but has been known to harm the liver or kidneys, in some patients.

After a great deal of consideration, Ashley refused traditional medicine. She was afraid the interferon would affect her organs and immune system. She was adamant about preferring natural treatments.

Carrie recommended a naturopathic doctor she had visited a few years earlier. This doctor herself had been treated and cured of multiple sclerosis, so she was the perfect choice for Ashley (more on this story later in the chapter).

At this point in her young life, Ashley was determined to heal. She went to the naturopath who recommended a complete detoxification, strict nutritional program, supplements, herbs, and an overall lifestyle change.

After a few months, Ashley began to improve. She was less tired, her muscles felt stronger, she looked healthier and felt pretty good, overall. She was diligent about her protocol, avoiding sweet, fried, processed, and inorganic foods, drinking lots of water, exercising, and otherwise taking better care of herself.

After several years, however, Ashley slowly slipped back into old habits. She got tired of the regimen, feeling it was too limiting. She went back to eating sugar, skipping her supplements, and not exercising. She had felt so well, she had forgotten what had happened to her, was in denial about having MS, and simply lived her life as she had before the diagnosis.

Ashley's body began a slow process of decline. Gradually, she lost muscle tone, balance, immunity, and a general feeling of wellness. It had taken Ashley four or five years of a fairly strict regimen to get healthy. After only a year of going off her protocol, her body had begun to slowly deteriorate.

At this point, Ashley had continued to refuse Western medicine to treat her MS, lost her will to maintain her holistic program, and had significantly given up. Negative emotional components and lack of intentional healing practices had also contributed to this decline, and her body responded by giving up on itself.

Today, fifteen years later, Ashley has a scooter that substitutes for her legs, and is on permanent disability. Yet, though her body is challenged, her spirits are high, she has maintained a strong faith and insists that she believes she'll heal. Ashley has maintained her sense of humor, receives physical therapy 3 times a week, and pays more attention to her nutrition. There is always hope, the development of new treatments and protocols, and the possibility of renewal and regeneration.

There are many stories, case studies, scientific evidence, and other reports of people healing from autoimmune disorders.

Holistic, integrative, or functional doctors know how to look at disease from the inside. Their methods, tools, training, treatments, protocols, and perspectives are very different from Western medical practices.

The natural perspective mandates that all diseases begin from inflammation, unhealthful nutrition, toxins, stress, and environment. Detoxification, particularly in the case of autoimmune diseases, is the first step (in most cases) toward healthy immunity.

CLAIRE

Claire had been ill for more than fifteen years with alternating symptoms of extreme fatigue, fever, swollen glands, depression, aching muscles, and overall weakness. These symptoms came and went for no apparent reason, sometimes for a day, other times for a week or longer. Yet, even during pain-free moments, there was consistently a low-grade malaise, and Claire struggled daily to maintain her life.

Claire was a physical therapist who needed energy and vitality to work properly. She worked every day, often feeling sick, tired, and discouraged. There were times when she needed to lean against a wall to support her body as she worked. She experienced such profound depression that thoughts of ending her life consumed her.

The doctors, who had no idea what was wrong with Claire, told her to rest, drink lots of fluids, and exercise lightly. This advice had become frustrating and useless very quickly, and Claire was desperate for answers. Constant fatigue and debilitation were daily companions, and Claire didn't know what to do.

After years of suffering with chronic illness, discomfort, frustration, and depression, she knew there had to be an answer, and was determined to feel better. Claire began to do research.

This was in 1987, when certain autoimmune diseases were still unknown. Chronic fatigue and Epstein-Barr virus were barely on the radar, usually diagnosed as cold or flu, with no protocol for treatment.

Around this time, Claire had remembered reading about an auto-immune disorder called Epstein-Barr Virus, and became convinced her symptoms matched those of this newly categorized virus. She told her general practitioner she wanted him to test her for it, at which point he told her the test was expensive and that there was no treatment for the virus, anyway. Claire encouraged him to test her in spite of it, and was determined to get a diagnosis in order to discover how to proceed. She had been learning about the effects of nutrition, supplements, and herbs on health, and was convinced she could find a solution.

The diagnosis turned up positive for the Epstein-Barr Virus, and Claire was both relieved and disturbed. What was she to do now that she had finally learned what the problem had been, after so many years of illness? Claire was determined to get well no matter what was involved, and whole-heartedly believed a cure was possible.

Claire had just begun a new job with a chiropractor, who was taking Chinese herbs and natural remedies for his own autoimmune disorder. Claire was hesitant to discuss her dilemma with him, for fear of losing her job, but decided the benefits of getting the proper care far outweighed the possibility of getting fired.

As it happened, the chiropractor told Claire about a Chinese herb-alist he had been seeing, and was convinced he could help her. Excited about the idea, she went to the herbal practitioner, who concurred with the diagnosis, and Claire began a long course of taking herbal remedies.

She also began a detoxification process to eliminate candida, heavy metals, and other toxins. Naturally, her body had been greatly compromised by toxins, chemicals, bacteria, and virus from many years of living in unhealthy environments, practicing poor nutrition, and being under tremendous stress.

Claire knew it wouldn't happen overnight, but at least she had significant indications of hope, and had always believed her body would heal, with the appropriate doctor and regimen. For the first time in years, Claire was able to trust a professional practitioner, and to see the light at the end of this long, dark tunnel.

Claire practiced yoga 3 times a week, deep breathing exercises daily, and went to the ocean weekly to rejuvenate her spirits. She attended a bi-weekly support group for women with similar disorders, and shared her story with others. Claire reached out to others who had experienced serious illnesses, and directed them to her own herbalist. She made a habit of practicing daily gratitude and envisioned her body in a state of optimum health.

Claire's medical doctor had told her that Epstein-Barr was incurable. Claire's story defies this belief system. It has now been almost thirty years since her diagnosis, and she is still well, thriving and healthy, with no signs or symptoms of the virus.

Claire had been sick for years, seeing doctor after doctor after doctor, with no diagnosis and no hope. After years of despair, she finally found the right practitioner at the right time, and was able to turn her illness into a success story.

MAX

Max had been diagnosed with stomach cancer in his early twenties. His doctor prescribed a series of chemotherapy treatments, which made Max very sick and weakened his immune system to the point where he experienced chronic infections. After the chemo, the doctors told Max his cancer was 90 percent gone, but they insisted on doing a few more rounds of chemo to try to eliminate the rest of the cancer.

Max decided not to do the additional treatments, and called on a friend to recommend a holistic alternative practitioner. Amanda, Max's friend, knew of a holistic medical doctor who had great success in treating various cancers, and Max was more than ready to meet him.

THIS HOLISTIC DOCTOR RECOMMENDED THE FOLLOWING PROTOCOLS:

- Detoxification
- Organic, specialized nutritional program
- Immune-enhancing supplements and herbs
- Hyperbaric oxygen therapy
- Intravenous vitamin and chelation therapies
- Positive attitude
- Visualization
- Cancer support group
- Meditation

Because Max's cancer had been very aggressive, he was advised to follow this protocol consistently and diligently—the effectiveness of the treatment was dependent on it, and it determined the speed with which his body would respond. There is no cancer treatment, whether it's holistic or medical, that is guaranteed, but it's important to consider that Max's regimen addressed the root or underlying causes of the disease, without ravaging his body.

This natural, alternative therapy was designed to support and boost Max's immune system while treating the cancer on a cellular level, without invasive therapy. The doctor also informed Max that his thoughts and emotions directly affected the health of his cells (this is true for all of us), and that the holistic approach to cancer was preferred and necessary.

Before doing any kind of treatment therapy, it's important to assess levels and amounts of toxic overload, nutritional deficiencies, immune-stressors, and absorption issues. To accomplish this, there are tests which include analysis of hair, urine, or blood, and other types of diagnostic equipment. These diagnostic tests will determine the therapies and supplements indicated for treatment. Max was given the entire evaluation before beginning his regimen.

MAX'S DETOXIFICATION AND NUTRITIONAL PROGRAM:
Pure alkaline water and appropriate nutrition are crucial to a successful anti-cancer strategy. Alkaline water creates an internal environment which cancer doesn't tolerate. Eating foods that support immunity while eliminating toxins, are highly effective in treating cancer, and knowing the foods that feed cancer are important to avoid, since they can interfere with the healing process.

Refined sugar feeds cancer cells and, in Max's case, was completely eliminated from his diet. Aspartame damages the body, as do refined flours and trans fatty acids. Dairy, processed foods, sodas, coffee, alcohol, and other chemicals cause inflammation in the body and might fuel the growth of cancer. A nutrient-rich diet enhances the healing process.

Max ate plant-based foods, which are nutritious and help the body eliminate toxins and heal. Fruits, vegetables, and herbs also cleanse and repair the body while inhibiting the growth of cancer. These include sea vegetables, leafy greens, broccoli, cabbage, cauliflower, dark grapes and berries, turmeric, ginger, garlic and green tea, and other antioxidants. Organic plant foods help protect the body from pathogenic invaders.

Olive oil and flaxseed oil need to remain unheated, while coconut oil can be used for cooking. Foods that enhance digestion are recommended, as opposed to large amounts of seeds and nuts, which slow down the process.

Max's diet consisted of very little animal protein, but his meats were only organic or grass-fed, including chicken and wild-caught fish. Beans and legumes are an important source of fiber, and Max ate them in moderation because some of them contain a few toxic elements.

He ate only gluten-free foods, since wheat and gluten contain sugar molecules, which overwhelm and clog digestion.

Foods and supplements such as chlorella, glutathione, milk thistle, mushroom extracts, glutamine, super antioxidants, super-green foods, zinc, selenium, propolis, andrographis, oregano oil, and elderflower have immune building properties and were, therefore, an integral part of Max's protocol. They also have cleansing properties, and therefore work synergistically to support immunity.

OXYGEN THERAPY:
Max received hyperbaric oxygen therapy treatments, since cancer is unable to survive in a highly oxygenated system. Other ways to deliver oxygen to the cells include exercise, deep breathing, ozone therapy, and alkaline water. Max received ozone therapy in a clinic in Mexico—there were not many, at the time, places in the United States for this particular treatment.

ALTERNATIVE CHEMOTHERAPY TREATMENTS:
These therapies are done together with all of the other treatments and protocols. Vitamin B17, or Laetrile, is found in apricot seeds, apples, and almonds, and targets only cancer cells. Max took this substance in Mexico, where it's legal, along with IP6 (a B-vitamin derivative), which also has anti-cancer properties.

LIFESTYLE:
Max received lymphatic drainage massages, acupuncture, got plenty of sleep, absorbed vitamin D3 from the sun, and exercised daily. He didn't eat at night, giving his liver the opportunity to work effectively. He also took coffee enemas for detoxification.

MEDITATION AND VISUALIZATION:
Max consciously attended to his spiritual growth through meditation and creative visualization, imagining himself healthy, vibrant, and cancer-free. He visualized eliminating toxic thoughts and emotions, and searched his soul to find self-love and compassion. Max joined a support group for his own emotional well-being, and to share stories with others who were dealing with cancer.

Although Max experienced moments of depression, fear, doubt, anger, frustration, and exhaustion, he alleviated his fears with the help of his family, friends, and entire holistic team.

Today, Max has been cancer-free for eighteen years, and lives a fulfilling and productive life. He has maintained his healthful lifestyle, gets lots of exercise, and practices meditation, gratitude, and yoga. He's a survivor who understands that his daily regimen, along with his diligence, literally, had saved his life.

JENNY

Jenny was a teenager with a serious sugar addiction. She consumed candy bars, cakes, chocolate, Twinkies, and ice cream in massive amounts. Her diet consisted of fast and fried foods, dairy, sodas, junk food, and generally everything unhealthy. Jenny was allowed to eat anything she wanted. This kind of diet was the perfect setup for immune deficiency, which eventually led to illness.

Jenny's mother and father had divorced when she was only three years old, and the feeling of loss of Mommy and Daddy together manifested itself into other problems. The stress of grief weighs heavily, especially on a young child. Jenny often felt anxious, fearful, insecure and unsafe.

Jenny had learned to manipulate the people, places, and things in her life to create an environment in which she felt in control. As she grew older, her unhealthful diet became a constant companion. Jenny's teeth were rotting from too much sugar, and dentists at that time used silver fillings made of mercury, known to cause neurological and physical disorders.

The toxins Jenny ingested and inhaled contributed to nightmares, trauma, and emotional instability. Her father's alcoholism was another factor. Jenny spent every other weekend with him, and when he was drunk, his criticism and abusive behavior were merciless. Jenny felt like a ping-pong ball, being shifted back and forth from one critical parent to the other.

Emotions, diet, trauma, criticism, and fear all contributed to the spiraling down of her health. Her immune system, at twenty-three, couldn't tolerate the weight of stress and an unhealthful diet, and Jenny experienced symptoms of Epstein-Barr virus and various other immune-deficient red flags. She had consistent symptoms of brain fog, fatigue, allergies, tightness in the chest, ear and sinus infections, sore throats, constipation, depression, weight loss, and dizziness.

Jenny's doctor recommended she get her brain and body checked by submitting to the following: MRI, EKG, urine sample, hearing test, and blood work. After all of the testing had been completed, surprisingly, everything came up negative. The doctors gave her shots and medicines, but nothing helped her feel better, and her symptoms continued to be chronic and debilitating.

Jenny's health had become more and more deficient as symptoms escalated, and she felt even more fearful as she began to lose her balance and speech. Out of desperation, Jenny's mother took her to a medical intuitive, a man who was able to see inside of disease. He told her that her body was full of candida, which had been caused by sugar, antibiotics, and the steroids the doctors had given her.

Jenny decided she'd had enough. Her life had become intolerable, and her resolve to heal was palpable. Jenny went home that day and furiously began her own research. She discovered that her disorientation had been caused from a by-product of candida called acetaldehyde, which becomes alcohol in the body and causes a feeling of being drunk. The more she learned the more she became determined to cure herself and continued to pursue solutions. The intuitive had recommended she take Nystatin, an antifungal that kills candida, and is plant based and non-toxic.

Jenny discovered, through her research, a food regimen that would kill off the fungal overgrowth, and after several months of changing her diet, was feeling better. Emotionally, however, Jenny was still addicted to dysfunctional relationships, negative thought patterns, and lack of spiritual connection. She had managed to change the physical aspects of her illness, but her emotional, mental, and spiritual beliefs had continued to jeopardize Jenny's overall condition.

At this time in her life, Jenny had moved several times from one place to another, believing that different locations would cure her. No matter where she moved, she couldn't maintain a job, and her negative feelings and thoughts continued to be pervasive.

After four years of an erratic lifestyle, bad choices and instability, Jenny had another attack of illness. She was sitting in a restaurant with a friend, and suddenly out of nowhere, she couldn't walk, speak, or think clearly. After a few minutes of panic, the paralysis ended, and Jenny was left, once again, with the disturbing realization that something was very wrong.

Lacking options, she was compelled to go home to her mother, who took her to see a neurologist. He tested her brain waves and sensory pathways. When the tests returned, Jenny was shocked to learn she had multiple sclerosis and that all of her symptoms over the past few years had been related to this disease. And by this time in her disease process, Jenny was confined to a wheel chair.

Upon hearing the diagnosis, Jenny felt a sense of heartbreak, confusion, and fear. When the neurologist told her chemotherapy (interferon) was the only known treatment for MS, Jenny was devastated. She had decided a few years back that she wasn't going to take medicine again because it had only made her feel worse; thus, interferon was not an option.

Multiple sclerosis is a disease of the central nervous system. Inflammation and toxins in the brain destroy the myelin sheath, which is a fatty tissue that protects the nerves. The myelin detaches from the nerves and becomes lesions (scar tissue) that forms over the sheath. The lesions can form in various parts of the brain and spinal cord, producing a multitude of symptoms.

Jenny decided to call the medical intuitive again, who told her to resume her healthful diet, take Nystatin, have the silver fillings in her mouth removed, and avoid sugar, alcohol, wheat, gluten, dairy and all inflammatory foods. He told her that if she followed his advice, she would completely heal, but that she must attack the disease from all sides—physically, mentally, spiritually, and emotionally.

Jenny was back on her regimen, taking daily Nystatin, omega fatty acids, and lots of vitamins C and E—long with a a full spectrum of vitamins and minerals, and ate only brown rice and vegetables. She knew it was crucial for her to clean house in all areas of her life, and began her healing process with the full intention of complete healing. It was a grueling, painstaking, frightening and lonely prospect, with consistent ocurrances of old demons, self-doubt, anxiety, rage, confusion, and other challenges.

Jenny worked hard on her sense of self-worth, confronting resistance and struggle all along the way. In a fit of hopelessness and despair when things weren't moving fast enough, Jenny considered taking her own life. However, she thought of her mother, who had sacrificed so much to help her, and changed her mind. The struggles and fears had continued to plague her for many, many months, even years, until very gradually, Jenny's life began to turn around.

A series of personal events, realizations, prayer, hypnotherapy, spiritual teachers, family support, self-awareness and a healthier attitude, became parts of Jenny's journey over the next few years, and, finally, her life changed dramatically.

All of Jenny's diligence, determination, understanding, and knowledge had made a difference. After having spent six or seven years with progressive deterioration and feelings of hopelessness, all the personal growth she had done served her well. Jenny was, once again, healthy, asymptomatic, and ready to take on the next phase of her life.

It's more than twenty-five years later, and Jenny is still healthy, thriving, and grateful, and has a wonderful life. She is a successful holistic practitioner, who helps many people with autoimmune diseases, especially multiple sclerosis.

If you suffer from MS and your doctor tells you that it's incurable, refer to Jenny's story and dare to take your own journey. It takes courage, conviction, and the right information to recover, against all odds.

There is no guarantee of healing, but the chances are much better with a holistic approach, which addresses the core issues of the disease.

NICOLE

Nicole and her husband had just moved into a house that was five-years old, a traditional home with a beautiful large backyard, fruit and avocado trees, and lots of space for their dogs. Nicole was living her dream.

After six months of living in the house, however, Nicole noticed a little patch of red, itchy bumps on her chest. She scratched them, didn't think much about it, and went on with her daily life. She consumed healthful foods, drank lots of water, ate dairy pretty regularly, drank a glass of wine now and then, exercised, and took care of herself (or at least she thought so).

Nicole was a photographer and got lots of sunshine and physical activity. She practiced yoga, meditation, pilates, received lymphatic massages, acupuncture and Reikii healings. She was living the good life and had a positive attitude, until at forty years old, it all began to change.

Nicole felt fatigued a lot of the time, developed allergies, began to get hot flashes and mood changes, and decided she was in the beginning of early menopause.

She made an appointment with her gynecologist, who confirmed Nicole was, indeed, premenopausal. Nicole wasn't happy to think she was experiencing this at such a young age, but according to the test results, it was undeniable. The gynecologist recommended she take bio-identical hormones to alleviate her symptoms, and, after a few months, Nicole had begun to feel a bit better. However, after several more months, her skin condition returned with a vengeance.

Nicole experienced more itching and had larger bump-like hives in clusters, which travelled around her body. They would appear out of nowhere, had lasted a few days or a week, and just as unexpectedly, they disappeared. The incidences had become more and more frequent, and the clusters were painful.

She didn't know what to do. Doctors and friends were perplexed, and even her gynecologist told her he had never seen this pattern before. He recommended Nicole see an allergist-friend of his, thinking it might be an allergic reaction to a food or something in the environment. Nicole went to the allergist, had allergy tests for different foods, grasses, flowers, trees, molds, chemicals, and other substances, and waited anxiously for the results.

The results arrived, and Nicole was surprised. Most of her allergies were to foods she rarely ate, as well as trees and grasses not native to where she lived. She discovered she was allergic to dust, feathers, cats, and hay, and had decided to have her house cleaned as frequently as possible. Nicole bought two air purifiers, putting one in her bedroom and the other in the living room. Several weeks later, however, she had still experienced painful, itchy hives, and was at a complete loss.

A friend suggested Nicole see an immunologist. Feeling as if she were out of other options, Nicole made the decision to see this doctor, who took a series of tests (blood panels), asked a lot of questions, and spent a lot of time with her. She was very thorough and professional, and Nicole was impressed with the doctor's manner. For the first time in many months, Nicole felt as if she were on the right track.

When the test results came back, Nicole discovered she was anemic, her thyroid count was low, and she had a few minor vitamin deficiencies. Surprisingly, she was in pretty good health. So why the rashes? The doctor prescribed vitamins, glandular Standard Process Brand (excellent quality product-line) for her thyroid, and an herbal combination supplement for her blood.

After several months, however, the rashes, pain, and other symptoms continued. By this time, Nicole was extremely disappointed, disheartened, and fearful that she would never find the answers. She had no idea what was happening to her, and didn't know where to turn.

She continued to take yoga classes to calm her breathing and mind, saw a Reiki master and another energy healer, did a week-long juice cleanse, and gave up the occasional glass of wine; but her symptoms remained. Her constant health-related battle created tensions between her and her husband, and Nicole had begun to feel as if life, as she had known it, was over.

One beautiful sunny day in Oregon, in Nicole's hometown, she was walking her dogs, when a neighbor she'd never met stopped to admire the dogs. The woman talked about animals, yoga, the neighbors, the school system, and general girl-talk. They discovered they had mutual friends, much in common, and had decided to meet for lunch the following week.

Nicole and Sandy met for lunch, talked and talked, and got to know one another. Nicole discovered Sandy was an integrative medical doctor, combining Western and alternative medicine in her practice. Nicole told Sandy about her symptoms, gave her the history of doctors she had seen, and expressed her frustration at not getting results from their recommendations. Sandy asked questions, was familiar with the kinds of symptoms Nicole had mentioned, and suggested Nicole come to her office the following day.

Sandy met Nicole in her office, asked more questions, did some muscle testing, and tested Nicole on a special machine that measures energy and heat waves in the body which indicate patterns of illness. Sandy evaluated that Nicole had large amounts of heavy metals, candida, and mold in her body, and deduced that these pathogens were causing her skin condition. Sandy suggested that Nicole and her husband have their house tested for mold.

Nicole and her husband, Peter, after having had their house tested for mold, were surprised to find out that underneath their bedroom floor boards, was a large amount of black mold, which is highly toxic and damages the immune system. Outraged because the house was only five years old, they decided to locate the builder and ask him how that could have happened. They also contacted the people who had sold them the house.

Nicole informed the builder about the mold, told him how sick she had been, and insisted he eliminate the flooring, clean out the mold, and put in new floors. After much resistance and denial, the builder finally admitted that the wood used in the bedrooms had been damaged by rain and hadn't dried properly. He shifted the blame to the architect for hiring incompetent carpenters. Nicole didn't care, at this point; she just wanted the job done immediately. Feeling the pressure from Nicole and Peter, the builder agreed to renovate the flooring at no cost. Nicole and Peter slept in a bedroom on the second floor of their house, until construction was completed.

In the meantime, Sandy recommended a chelation therapy intravenous drip treatment (eliminates heavy metals), along with glutathione and antioxidants in her diet for detoxification—one chelation treatment weekly for ten to twenty weeks. In addition, she prescribed several other supplements, minerals, and herbs to completely cleanse Nicole's body. Sandy also suggested Nicole do a green juice fast for two days to begin the process, and outlined a very specific diet for post-detoxification.

After a month of detoxification, Nicole began to feel better, had less skin problems, and had more energy and vitality. She continued with the treatments, was diligent about her nutrition, and felt better and better as time passed. She completed the ten chelation treatments, and by the end of the ten weeks and after a long and difficult personal journey, Nicole had successfully returned to her naturally healthy self.

This is another classic example of healing from toxins and illness with the proper diagnosis, doctor, and treatments. It was serendipity that Nicole and Sandy had met at a time when Nicole was in dire need of answers.

This scenario is a characteristic dilemma for people with autoimmune disorders—too many doctors and not enough answers. In Nicole's case, the results were significantly triumphant, and she was able to resume her normal life. Nicole's attitude about healing, her emotional and spiritual practices—yoga, pilates, meditation, acupuncture, working with a Reikii healer—all of these holistic aspects had contributed to Nicole's healing process.

SAM

Sam had been a dentist for over thirty years at a time when dentists stood on their feet for hours in a day. The dental equipment was different from what it is today, and dentists rarely sat on stools, like they do now. Sam had severe back and leg problems as a result, and, over time, the veins in his legs had become varicose.

Sam was in his seventies and retired when he was diagnosed with prostate cancer. In addition, Sam had experienced atrial fibrillations (heart palpitations) for most of his life, having had scarlet fever as a young boy. He also had an enlarged heart. The irony of it was that for most of his life, Sam had been healthy, rarely having colds, flu, or any kind of illness. He had lived a good life, travelled to many countries with his wife, had three wonderful children and great friends, and was a loving, generous, and endearing man.

When confronting prostate cancer, Sam's oncologist gave him a few options: remove the prostate, chemotherapy, or female hormones, which inactivate the gland so that the cancer has little opportunity to grow. Prostate cancer is normally slow-growing in older men, and therefore, less likely to metastasize or cause death.

Sam chose the hormone therapy treatment rather than invasive chemotherapy. He was aware of the trajectory of this kind of cancer in an older man, and decided to treat it as naturally as possible. His son-in-law, a holistic medical doctor, prescribed massive doses of antioxidants, such as vitamins C, E, B12, D and A, mineral supplements, and super-nutrient foods and herbs.

Sam was diligent about his supplements and got plenty of exercise, in spite of chronic pain in his back, knees, and legs. He had taken good care of himself, and because of his diligence, his cancer didn't grow, spread, or cause any significant problems. The doctors had been more concerned about his heart, atrial fibrillations, bad circulation and severe varicose veins.

Sam's son-in-law had suggested a series of chelation therapies to remove the plaque from his arteries. In addition, Sam had high cholesterol and erratic blood pressure, which relates to blockages in the arteries. At that time, in his late seventies, Sam had slowed down a bit, and was certainly confronted with his own mortality.

Sam, in spite of his age and Western medical education, had been a great champion of alternative medicine, had great faith in his son-in-law, and decided chelation therapy was appropriate for him. Sam willingly completed the series of treatments-- typically twenty in all-- and the results proved to be well worth the effort.

The process of chelation therapy requires patience, usually consisting of four hours of intravenous vitamins, minerals, and natural substances, during which time one can read, sleep, eat, drink lots of water, talk with others in treatment, or sit and meditate. The intravenous drip is administered gradually and methodically by a professional who is trained, licensed, and competent, and the patient is monitored throughout the protocol. The entire course of treatment can take anywhere from twenty weeks to several months, depending on the prescription.

The doctor takes X-rays of the heart and arteries before and after the procedures; in Sam's case, the results were successful and quite possibly, lifesaving. Sam's heart had been compromised from years of enlargement, fibrillations, and a significant buildup of plaque. Chelation therapy, most likely, had added years to his life.

Because of Sam's age, the cancer had almost no chance of causing a serious problem, whereas his heart had been more likely to be a culprit, after so many years of damage.

There are numerous case studies, individual studies, and scientific evidence which indicate that chelation is highly effective and has saved lives. The practice is also implemented more and more frequently by integrative, functional medical doctors and practitioners.

In a review of forty published and unpublished studies involving over twenty-five thousand patients who had undergone chelation therapy, an 87 percent success rate was reported by those who benefited from the treatment.

Chelation therapy works intravenously with a powerful antioxidant called ethylenediaminetetraacetic acid (EDTA). This substance enters the bloodstream and attaches onto heavy metals such as mercury, cadmium, lead, excess calcium, arsenic, and other damaging chemicals, and eliminates them from the body through urine.

Calcification in the arteries is a major cause of atherosclerosis, and chelation is a method which functions to increase blood flow and discourage the formation of blood clots, which can be potentially life-threatening. It also reduces the pain of angina. It's estimated that in the past fifty years or so, millions of people have undergone this therapy for a wide range of problems, and chelation has an extremely good record of safety.

There are many, many patients who are alive and well, and avoided invasive surgeries like angioplasty, bypass, and stents—Sam was one of them.

For the next five or six years, Sam continued to live an active life until age eighty-five, when he fell and broke his hip. His varicose veins, without treatment, had become more serious. While recovering from hip surgery, a vein in one of his legs burst, and because he had been taking Coumadin, a blood thinner, Sam bled out and, sadly, passed away.

It's quite possible that had Sam not taken the Coumadin, which had thinned his blood, he might have survived. The chelation therapy had significantly reduced his chances of a heart attack, according to his medical records and several doctors, and the hormone treatment had controlled his cancer, but nothing could have controlled the vein that burst in his leg.

If you had asked Sam, who had experienced significant amounts of pain daily in those last years, he had been ready to pass on. He would have told you how wonderful his life had been, that he had lived with no regrets, and that he had been ready to go on to his next journey.

PHILIP

Philip was only twelve-years old when his sister, Megan, died of leukemia at age fifteen. This had been a severely traumatic event for Philip, who, at that time, was a budding adolescent and adored his sister. They were close siblings and had spent lots of time riding bikes, hiking, dancing, and playing board games. Megan had studied ballet since age four, and one of Philip's favorite pastimes was watching her dance.

When Megan passed away after a year of chemotherapy, radiation, hospital visits, and a great deal of other invasive treatments that had made her very ill, Philip went into a deep depression. His parents were experiencing their own grief, and didn't have the knowledge or understanding to deal with Philip's feelings. As a consequence, Philip moped around the house, overate, slept too much, and wasn't getting good grades in school.

A family friend, Paul, who was a pediatrician, suggested Philip see a psychologist who could encourage him to talk about his feelings. It took many sessions before Philip opened up to Dr. Collins, but gradually he was able to share his feelings, cry, and talk about his sister, Megan.

Dr. Collins suggested Philip enroll in a dance class, an activity that might prove to be therapeutic. After much convincing, Philip joined a ballet class, just as his sister had many years before. At first he hated it, thinking it was only for girls, and didn't pay much attention in class. But little by little, as he became more limber and adept, he began to enjoy the movement. The joy he felt while dancing motivated him to want to lose weight, and he made that his mission. Philip became obsessed with his weight loss-- running daily, subsisting on only watermelon and almonds, and refusing to eat anything else.

His behavior was unusually compulsive, indicating symptoms of obsessive-compulsive disorder (OCD). Phyllis and John, his parents, still oblivious to Philip's erratic behavior, simply thought Philip had been in a "phase," and would eventually come out of it.

After a year or so, Philip's eating habits hadn't changed, and he still exhibited signs of OCD, but had added other foods to his diet: a variety of nuts, seeds, fruits, and chocolate. His parents and Dr. Collins were concerned, doing everything they could to reason with him. But the more they talked, the less he paid attention. Philip was annoyed with the constant pressure to eat differently and finally refused to see Dr. Collins at all, insisting he was fine and didn't need her. He was unreasonably stubborn, implacable, and relentless. Philip maintained that he had become vegan because he loved animals too much to eat them, and persisted with his diet of choice.

By the time he was fifteen, Philip's behavior was out of control. He exhibited behavioral mood swings and temper tantrums, couldn't concentrate in school, and had few friends. This had become progressively worse over the course of several years, and Philip's parents finally relented and called Dr. Collins to ask her if she would make a house call.

Dr. Collins came to the house, talked with a reluctant Philip for as long as she could keep his attention, and diagnosed that he was exhibiting symptoms of manic depression, or bipolar disorder. His parents, of course, were shocked. They had denied, for so many years, that anything other than growing pains had been the problem, and this news took them completely by surprise. Dr. Collins, adamant about immediate treatment, prescribed medication for Philip.

By the third week of taking the prescription, however, Philip had decided he hated the medication because it made him feel fuzzy and listless, interfered with his dancing, and refused to take it.

Phyllis and John, at this point, were faced with a serious dilemma— what to do, and how to cope with Philip's difficult and inconsistent behavior. Their friend, Paul, who had recommended Dr. Collins, as a last resort, suggested Philip see an integrative medical doctor. Paul conjectured that perhaps Philip was deficient in vitamins and minerals due to his limited food choices, and might benefit from a more balanced diet.

Blood tests revealed Philip's body chemistry was seriously depleted, that the teenager's vitamin and mineral counts resembled that of a fifty-year-old. His thyroid was out of the normal range and hormone levels very low for his age, as well as severe deficiencies in other areas.

It was no wonder he exhibited mood swings and obsessive-compulsive behavior. Philip's body was aging more rapidly than that of a healthy fifteen-year-old, and he was unable to focus, sit still, or listen to his teachers. Dance was the only healthy activity Philip engaged in joyfully, diligently, and consistently. He was able to express all of his emotions through dance, and loved it passionately.

Dr. Stephens, the recommended integrative medical doctor, was an affable man, had a great sense of humor, loved ballet, and managed to make a connection with Philip that no one else had been able to. Philip respected him, listened to him, and had decided that this doctor was his kind of guy— a man who didn't force him to take medications, but rather, gave him suggestions and alternatives for a healthful, balanced, and nutrient-rich diet.

Philip began a regimen of high doses of antioxidants, multi-minerals, probiotics, and powdered super-nutrient rich foods, along with lots of healthy protein and supplements prescribed to reduce anxiety and depression.

THIS IS A PARTIAL LIST OF PHILIP'S TREATMENT PROTOCOL:

- Protandim
- Q96
- Bacopa
- Ashwagandha
- Milk thistle
- Green tea
- Turmeric
- Hops
- 5-HTP
- Passion flower
- L-Theanine
- Lemon balm
- Lavender baths
- Chamomile tea

These herbs and spices helped reduce Philip's inflammation, toxicity, blood sugar, liver function, and anxiety and depression.

Because Philip was also diagnosed with mold, heavy metals, candida, and other pathogenic toxins, Dr. Stephens prescribed a detoxification program in addition to:

- Vitamins A, C, D and E
- Thiamine
- Riboflavin
- Niacin
- B6
- Folic acid
- Biotin
- Pantothenic acid
- Iron
- Iodine
- Grape-seed extract
- Glutamine
- Glutathione
- L-Methionine
- Ginkgo biloba
- Germanium
- Boron
- Phenylalanine
- Citrus bioflavonoids
- Choline

THE VITAMINS AND MINERALS IN THESE SUPPLEMENTS COMPLETED THE BENEFICIAL EFFECTS IN THE FOLLOWING WAYS:

- Mood and brain function support
- Support and cleansing of all bodily systems
- Immunity building
- Preventative factors

- Calming agents
- High antioxidant levels
- Richness in micronutrients, which are easily absorbed and utilized
- Excellent bioavailability for digestion

After two years of a proper diet and this particular supplemental protocol, Philip, now seventeen, felt better than he ever had, maintained a healthy weight, and exhibited less signs of OCD and bipolar disorder.

Dr. Stephens's protocols had been successful in turning Philip's life around. Philip had begun to experience more clarity and focus, while feeling less anxious and depressed, and had a much longer attention span. The diet and supplements had given Philip's body more balance, and by this time, his mood swings and obsessions had almost disappeared.

Phillip had decided, in honor of his sister, to use his considerable dance and athletic skills to audition for a reputable ballet company. After several auditions, Philip was accepted into the company, and was well on his way to achieving his dream.

There are, of course, hereditary components involved in chemical imbalances which affect the emotions, and sometimes pharmaceutical medications are indicated. At the same time, the most knowledgeable practitioners support evidence that heredity can be altered, as can DNA, with the proper and appropriate nutritional supplements.

There are thousands of stories like these-- stories about healing autoimmune diseases and mental illnesses with natural remedies.

There will always be doubters, doctors who think it's all speculative and, worse, pharmaceutical companies that would lose billions of dollars if people stopped taking medicine.

It takes courage, faith, patience, spiritual and emotional practices which infiltrate into our cells and DNA, and a professional support system, in order to "go natural." Since autoimmune diseases can be healed under the right circumstances, it's imperative that you educate yourselves to read, learn, do the research, talk to people who are knowledgeable and informed, and investigate your options. It might very well be the decision that saves or changes your life.

CHAPTER 5

CANCER: UNCOMMON PROTOCOLS, NUTRITION, HERBS AND SUPPLEMENTS

Uncommon protocols, nutrition, herbs and supplements are crucially important elements in effectively treating cancer. Once the body is completely detoxified, even in third and fourth-stage cancer— and this might be a delicate but supervised process, it's essential to rebuild and nourish the immune system with super-nutrients, powerful herbs, antioxidants and natural, alternative protocols.

Many integrative, holistic, and alternative doctors work exclusively with cancer patients and are highly qualified to recommend a comprehensive protocol. The number of patients who've been cured from even fourth-stage cancer is worthy of note.

Scientific and innovative research, treatments, and information have reached transformative levels. People have been, and continue to be, cured—meaning, so far, in complete remission, asymptomatic and without tumors or active cancer cells. The cases which are particularly significant are those patients who have remained healthy for 15 or more years, and there are many.

FOODS

Foods and nutritional choices are particularly important in treating cancer. Because cancer can't survive in an alkaline environment, alkaline foods and liquids are highly recommended.

Here is a partial list of alkaline foods:

VEGETABLES

- Alfalfa
- Beet greens
- Broccoli
- Cabbage
- Carrot
- Cauliflower
- Chard green
- Chlorella
- Cucumber
- Dandelion
- Garlic
- Green bean
- Green pea
- Kale
- Lettuce
- Mustard green
- Onion
- Parsley
- Pepper
- Pumpkin
- Radish
- Spirulina
- Sprouts
- Sweet potato
- Watercress
- Wheatgrass

FRUITS

- Apple
- Apricot

- Avocado
- Banana
- Berry
- Cantaloupe
- Cherry (sour)
- Coconut
- Currant
- Date
- Fig
- Grape
- Lemon
- Lime
- Nectarine
- Peach
- Pear
- Pineapple
- Raisin
- Raspberry
- Rhubarb
- Strawberry
- Watermelon

PROTEIN

- Almond
- Cashew
- Chestnut
- Millet
- Quinoa
- Tempeh
- Tofu

If meats or poultry are consumed, they must be organic and grass-fed, lean and from reliable sources, are not alkaline in nature. Fatty meats are not recommended.

GRAINS AND LEGUMES

- Brown rice
- Buckwheat
- Quinoa
- Soy beans

SEEDS

- Black seed
- Caraway seed

EAT RIGHT

The urge to cheat, which we all experience, is not only a physical response, but also an emotional and psychological reaction to stress and imbalance. Before you react to a craving or desire, think of the consequences. If you have an autoimmune disorder, particularly cancer, a healthful, well-balanced diet is essential to healing.

Organic foods are also highly recommended. Increasingly, grocery stores are stocking organic products because of the need and demand for them. Organic products are easily available, and are, in some stores, inexpensive.

People around the country are growing their own foods, as organic farming on personal property, parks, and homesteads is becoming the new paradigm in farming. Many farmers sell their fruits and vegetables at local farmers' markets.

Along with healthful eating, it's recommended to take regular antioxidants, like vitamin C, D3, B complex, E, A, and K2, as well as a multi-mineral complex, and a high-content probiotic supplement to maintain balance in the gut. Inflammation is a significant component of cancer, and alkalinizing foods are your best friend, as is oxygenating the body.

SUPPLEMENTS, HERBS, AND UNCOMMON TREATMENTS FOR CANCER:

BLACK SEED OIL AND THYMOQUINONE

Black "cumin" seed oil is an herb found mostly in countries around the Mediterranean Sea and India. It's known to be a potent herb used to heal a variety of pathogenic agents—most significantly, cancer. Black seed oil inhibits cancer cell activity and possibly kills specific types of cancer cells. Scientific research in animal studies has shown that black seed oil (Nigella sativa) is an effective treatment for cancer. "Studies show that black seed oil is as effective as anticancer drugs for certain types of cancer."

Black cumin seed oil and its extract, thymoquinone, have powerful benefits for various inflammatory cancers, including liver, melanoma (skin), pancreatic, cervical, breast, bone, stomach, lymphoma, prostate, colon, and brain cancers.

Despite several decades of extensive private research on black seed oil for treating cancer, pharmaceutical research companies have rarely advanced the work into human clinical testing, even though the benefits are dynamic and the risks of negative side effects have proven to be extremely low.

In individual cases and numerous case studies, black seed oil for cancer prevention and treatment has proven to be a powerful strategy. In two separate studies, Chinese researchers and Saudi Arabian researchers reviewed the scientific literature for the use of black seed oil in treating cancer. They both supported and substantiated the anticancer properties of this safe and natural seed oil. They emphasized that black seed oil has been used in their countries as a traditional medicine for centuries. The oil and its extracted component, thymoquinone, are both effective against many other diseases, including cardiovascular disease, diabetes, asthma, and kidney disease.

The researchers indicated that, although the molecular structures behind thymoquinone's anticancer role are not clearly understood, some studies showed that it's also a powerful antioxidant, improves the body's immune system, and induces apoptosis (the body's ability to eliminate unhealthy cells) without releasing toxins into the bloodstream.

Although the anticancer properties of black seed were recognized thousands of years ago, in the past two or three decades, modern scientific research has now been undertaken to study this valuable oil for use in traditional medicine.

Considering the positive and curative effects of black seed on a variety of pathogens, there is hope that our medical and pharmaceutical communities continue to get up to speed with this substance, and with other successful holistic healing methods.

Egyptian researchers studied the protective effect of bee honey and black seeds on cancer by exposing rats to a strong carcinogen. After four groups of rats were exposed to the cancer-causing agent, three groups were fed either black seeds or honey, while one group was fed both. The rats were then evaluated after six months. Those that ate black seeds received 80 percent protection against cancer-causing cells. The rats that ate only honey received no significant benefit, except they went back for more. The rats that ate a daily dose of both honey and black seeds were protected 100 percent against inflammatory responses and cancer growth.

In a 2014 study, Turkish researchers reported that black seed oil could potentially be helpful to people who are receiving radiation treatment for cancer. This study investigated the effects of radiation and the addition of black seed oil on the liver tissue of radiated rats. Researchers exposed rats to a single dose of radiation. One study group of rats received one gram of black seed oil per kilogram of body weight one hour before radiation, and a daily dose afterward for ten days. Another group received radiation treatment and was given a saline solution instead of black seed oil. The analysis of the data showed the black seed oil increased the antioxidant activity in the liver tissue of rats. The evidence showed that the use of black seed oil before radiation, and for ten days afterward, protected the rats from some of the harmful side effects of radiation.

A scientific study in Saudi Arabia investigated the anticancer activity of black seed oil and black seed extract when used to treat human lung cancer cells in a laboratory. Scientists exposed lung cancer cells to black seed oil or to black seed extract for twenty-four hours. They used 0.01 mg/ml to 1 mg/ml of the oil or extract, and after exposure, the cancer cells were evaluated.

Results showed both the black seed oil and extract significantly reduced cancer cells and changed the cellular composition of the tumors. Scientists found that the greater the concentration of the oil or extract used, the greater the level of cancer cell death. Researchers concluded that black seed extract and oil significantly reduced the proliferation of human lung cancer cells.

Researchers from Ohio State University published a study in 2013 noting that glioblastoma, or brain cancer, is the most aggressive and common type of malignancy in humans, with an average survival rate of fifteen months.

Phytochemicals have received much scientific attention because many exhibit potent anticarcinogenic action. Thymoquinone, one of the bioactive compounds of black seed oil, has antioxidant, anti-inflammatory and anticancer actions; it also kills human cancer cells without causing harm to normal cells.

The Ohio State University study examined how thymoquinone selectively inhibits the ability of glioblastoma cancer cells of the brain and spinal cord from replicating. This phytochemical also inhibits the continued growth of cancer cells. The result is a regression of tumor progression and extended survival of organs affected by tumors.

A 2013 study conducted in Malaysia addressed the anticancer properties of thymoquinone when used for long-term treatment of human breast cancer. It showed a sustained ability to inhibit breast cancer cell growth. The length of inhibition provided by this process was determined by the size of the dose—larger doses produced more significant results.

The same kinds of studies were conducted on a variety of cancers, including leukemia, colon, liver, and kidney. The results were similar, with minor variations. The black seed and thymoquinone effectively reduced both the size and amount of cancer cells in the organs and blood. Apoptosis, which is cancer cell death, was indicated in all of these studies.

In 2010, Saudi Arabian researchers noted that a large number of diseases are attributed to Helicobacter pylori (H. pylori), including chronic active gastritis, peptic ulcer disease, and gastric cancer (gut/immunity connection). H. pylori's resistance to antibiotics is increasing, and it's necessary to find effective treatment. Black seeds possess excellent anti-helicobacter properties and have been used to treat the bacteria, with very positive results.

A researcher from Oman, an Arab country, states the obvious fact—that thymoquinone oil has been extensively studied. The use of this substance with human cancer cells and in animal studies (with induced forms of cancer) has been thoroughly investigated. The result is that a considerable amount of information was generated, thus providing a better understanding of the antiproliferating properties of this supplement. It's appropriate, therefore, to encourage more global clinical trials to be conducted on this remarkable compound, and for medical and pharmaceutical industries to take it more seriously.

GLUTATHIONE

GHS, or glutathione, which is called "the master builder," is an important antioxidant that builds cells, detoxifies heavy metals in the blood, and is antiaging. It's a miraculous and powerful resource because it plays a crucial role in treating a variety of diseases:

- Aids
- Alzheimer's
- Cancer

- Crohn's
- Chronic Fatigue
- Dermatitis
- Diabetes
- Down Syndrome
- Heart Disease
- Glaucoma
- Hair and Hearing Loss
- Huntington's Chorea
- Hepatitis
- High Cholesterol
- Inflammatory Bowel Disease
- Kidney Failure
- Lung Disease
- Macular Degeneration
- Male Infertility
- Multiple Sclerosis
- Pancreatitis
- Parkinson's Disease
- Prostate Problems
- Psoriasis
- Schizophrenia
- Stroke

INTRAVENOUS GLUTATHIONE:
Glutathione is an important antioxidant for the entire body, including the brain. Intravenous glutathione has been used as a complementary treatment for cancer, heavy metal overload, environmental illness, and a host of autoimmune diseases, including Parkinson's.

Glutathione and other enzymes are depleted in an area of the brain called the "substantia nigra," in patients with Parkinson's. The primary function of glutathione is to protect the body's cells from oxidative stress. Glutathione enhances the function of other antioxidant compounds by keeping them stabilized and by eliminating pathogens from the body.

In 1996, it was reported that a group of Italian researchers were given glutathione twice a day for one month. The results were highly significant, as they exhibited improvement of various kinds of immune deficiencies. Perhaps even more impressive, was that after the treatment ended, the therapeutic effect lasted for as long as two to four months.

Another study from Japan in 1984 reported that glutathione can be an effective treatment for liver cancer. A trial of six patients with liver cancer on 5 g of oral glutathione daily (amount of time varies from one patient to the next), found reduction or arrestment of tumor growth in three of them. One patient had a reduction in "alpha-fetoprotein" (a tumor marker) from 496 to 5. Two of the six patients survived for one year.

Statistics of various treatments of this substance have indicated that how often glutathione can be administered to a patient, depends on the doctor's evaluation and recommendation. It's also dependent on the type and stage of the cancer.

The usefulness of glutathione as an anti-tumor agent might be limited so far to the liver, kidney, and peripheral neurons because, so far, these are the only tissues able to transport glutathione for cellular absorption.

A pilot trial with forty-five participants was reported to investigate the effect of glutathione on the side-effects of radiation therapy. Patients were given 1200 mg of glutathione, or a saline placebo, intravenously fifteen minutes prior to pelvic radiation. Patients receiving glutathione suffered less from post-radiation diarrhea and were more likely to complete the treatment cycle. There was evidence of greater tumor reduction in the glutathione group—73 percent—compared to 62 percent in the control group.

Another trial reportedly studied the neuro-protective effect of intravenous glutathione (1500 mg/m2) during chemotherapy treatment for gastric cancer. After nine weeks of treatment, no patient of the twenty-four receiving glutathione had neuropathy symptoms. Meanwhile, sixteen of eighteen patients who received the placebo experienced numbness and pain.

A trial of seventy-nine women with ovarian cancer found that intravenous administration of 2500 mg glutathione prior to che-motherapy, led to greater tumor response and reduced over-all toxicity, compared to that found in other trials using only chemotherapy.

Glutathione is a powerhouse antioxidant with a multitude of heal-ing elements. It's important to make it a part of your daily regi-men, especially if you have cancer or experience toxic overload.

These results are highly significant and mandate the implementa-tion of more broad-spectrum research.

IP6 SUPPLEMENT

The anticancer effects of IP6 are well worth noting. Research shows that in addition to reducing cancer cell growth, IP6 might restore cancerous cells back to their normal state. Also known as inositol hexaphosphate or phytic acid, IP6 is a sugar molecule with six phosphate molecules attached. It's composed of inositol, B vita-min, and six molecules of phosphorous. IP6 has only recently been researched as both a preventative treatment and cure for liver cancer, heart disease, kidney stones, Parkinson's disease, and more. It's reported to be a powerful antioxidant and immune booster, and has the capability to transform cancer cells.

Foods that are significant sources of IP6 include: dried beans, wheat germ, wheat bran, cereals, whole grains, nuts, seeds, rice, corn, and sesame.

It has been reported that a scientist from the University of Maryland Medical School did extensive research on IP6, beginning his work in the late 1980s. He discovered the ability of IP6 to control cancer cell division long after cancer was induced. His research indicated that IP6 normalized the sugar production of cancerous cells (sugar feeds cancer cells), thereby altering the component toward a healthier state. The ability of IP6 to change the structure of cancer cells has significant implications, since cancer cells that are controlled are less harmful to the body.

The study indicates that the value of IP6 lies in its ability to directly affect the physiology of cancerous cells. The research focused on controlling cancer to a point at which normal cells were restored.

BENEFITS OF IP6:
Normalizes the Rate of Cell Growth- Cancer cells have no control over dividing too rapidly and having a devastating impact on health. IP6 normalizes the rate at which cancer cells divide.

Helps Normalize Cell Physiology- How a cancer cell expresses itself largely determines its level of threat. Experiments show that IP6 has the ability to alter the chemistry of a cancer cell, thereby impacting its toxic effect.

Enhances NK ("natural killer") Cells- These are white blood cells that help protect against cancerous cells. Research indicates that the higher the NK activity, the lower the incidence of some cancers. A healthy human being produces five hundred to one thousand cancer cells daily. NK cells and apoptosis (cell death) result in the destruction and removal of a large number of these cells. Stress interferes with NK activity, which is why there's a direct connection between stress and cancer. IP6 increases NK cells during times of stress.

Increases Tumor Suppressor p53 Gene Activity- DNA contains tumor suppressor genes that inhibit cancer cell growth. The p53 gene prevents cancerous cells from growing and propagating. If the p53 gene becomes damaged or compromised, cancer can establish itself more readily. IP6 has been proven to increase the amount of p53 gene activity up to seventeen times its normal rate of activity.

Reduces Inflammation- The level of systemic inflammation is an important indicator in determining the outcome of cancer. Inflammation results in the release of cytokines, which are chemical messengers that trigger reactions that enable normal cells to grow and repair themselves. IP6 significantly reduces inflammation by stimulating healthy cytokines in the cells.

Potent Antioxidant- Antioxidants protect against various diseases and aging. They prevent free radicals and oxidation from damaging the body. This allows oxygenation to flow through the body, thus stimulating cells, blood and circulation. Damage to DNA leaves cells susceptible to mutation, resulting in the growth of cancerous cells. IP6 protects the body from damage.

Enhances Apoptosis- Programmed cell death, known as apoptosis, results in the removal of cancerous cells without affecting surrounding healthy cells. In a healthy body, apoptosis usually occurs when cells are damaged. IP6 helps remove damaged cells which cause inflammation.

Affects Angiogenesis- Angiogenesis is the process by which tumors set up their own blood supply, supplying the nutrients necessary to fuel their growth. Once the blood supply is formed, tumor growth increases as more proliferation leads to more blood supply. IP6 inhibits angiogenesis, resulting in cutting off the blood supply to cancer cells.

Inhibits Metastasis- IP6 inhibits the adhesion of cancer cells to proteins, leading to reduced cell migration and invasion (certain cancers are protein-receptive). Limiting adhesion is very important after surgeries and biopsies, which can cause cancer cells to metastasize.

One reason so many breast cancer patients are found to have lymph nodes containing cancer cells is that mammography can dislodge cancer cells, which then move to the lymph nodes.

Ask your gynecologist about thermography, a more effective way to detect breast cancer because there's no radiation involved and it's a non-invasive, painless procedure. The process is done by infrared imaging, known to detect cancer ten years before the capability of a mammogram.

Poly-MVA

Another important supplement, Poly-MVA, is a complex combination of minerals, vitamins, and amino acids designed to support cellular energy production and promote overall health. It replaces specific nutrients depleted during chemotherapy or radiation. Poly-MVA is a breakthrough supplement that assists in boosting the immune response and supports damaged cells. It contains a combination of alpha-lipoic acid and palladium, vitamins B1, B2, B12, formylmethionine, n-acetyl cysteine, and trace amounts of molybdenum, rhodium, and ruthenium. Poly-MVA targets the "energy charge transfer mechanism" of the cells and protects them from free radicals. It's completely safe, multifaceted, and extremely beneficial for optimum health, and protects DNA and RNA as it neutralizes free radicals.

The first report of clinical studies of Poly-MVA was presented in March 1994 by the late Dr. Rudolf E. Falk, an oncologist and surgeon at the University of Toronto. Dr. Falk stated that Poly-MVA was administered intravenously to ninety-five cancer patients. These included diagnoses of breast, lung, colorectal, prostate, pancreatic, ovarian, malignant melanoma, and primary brain cancers. 90 percent of the patients were in the category of having failed all conventional therapy, such as chemotherapy and radiation. Eighty-eight percent were surviving on only chemotherapy with a projected survival rate of nine months. The projected survival time of this group would vary from 20 percent to 60 percent in six months, depending on the stage of the cancer.

The first twenty-seven patients given Poly-MVA were considered terminal, and all had refused to continue with conventional chemotherapy. Their particular cancers involved tongue, lung, breast, esophagus, stomach, colon, pancreas, brain, prostate, lymph, blood, and bone marrow, and all had metastasized. They were initially given five drops of Poly-MVA four times daily. Thirteen reported improved appetites, weight gain, increased energy, and pain reduction within the first seven days of starting Poly-MVA. At the end of fourteen days, six additional patients reported improvement. None of the twenty-seven patients reported adverse reactions.

Another study reported that a seventy-five-year-old female with glioblastoma (brain cancer), and a history of surgeries, was given two complete rounds of radiation and tamoxifen chemotherapy.

After the treatment, her memory was impaired, she required help walking, and her speech was slurred.

On the third day after beginning Poly-MVA, her memory and speech improved, but she lived for only six months. Physical evidence indicated that her immediate death was attributed to the side effects of the tamoxifen, which she had continued to take before and after the Poly-MVA. The rounds of chemotherapy and radiation had destroyed her immune system, and her body was unable to fight off opportunistic pathogens.

In another case, a female patient experienced pain and inflammation from metastatic breast cancer of the spine and right hip. She had required a right hip replacement, which gave her relief from hip pain, but did not address the spinal cancer. The patient began Poly-MVA and within two weeks, her back pain stopped and she returned to her job.

In yet another case study, two patients with cancer of the esophagus had been suffering from cachexia (starvation) and were terminal when they began Poly-MVA. One patient was in a hospital when he was scheduled to begin the Poly-MVA. The other patient took the Poly-MVA at home. The first patient died within six weeks, but an investigation uncovered the fact that he had never been given the Poly-MVA; he had been given only Laetrile (B17). The second patient reported increased strength and weight gain, and was still alive two years after having taken Poly-MVA.

ORGANIC GERMANIUM

Germanium is a trace mineral cited as one of the greatest new developments in the natural treatment of cancer. In its inorganic form, germanium has no nutritional benefit. Inorganic germanium is related to silicon, and is used in the electronics industry to make computer chips.

However, organic geranium, also called germanium-132, or GeOxy-132, has been known to protect the body from cancer and tumor growth by strengthening the immune system. Germanium is also a potential treatment for cancer and other degenerative diseases associated with aging and free-radical damage.

Many important herbs and medicinal plants traditionally used in healing, including ginseng, garlic, comfrey, and aloe, all contain substantial amounts of germanium. It's estimated that the therapeutic benefits of these herbs might be linked to their high amounts of organic germanium.

A Japanese doctor was the first to successfully create organic germanium. He discovered that it protects against cancer by stimulating the production of interferon, a substance that stimulates the production of natural killer cells, which combat cancer. This doctor was the first to develop the process for producing an organic germanium, chemically identical to the form extracted from plants. The chemical name for this organic germanium compound is "bis-carboxyethyl germanium sesquioxide." Organic germanium helps increase oxygen in the body, slowing the growth of cancer cells and helping them return to their natural state.

Cancer cells cannot survive in an oxygen-rich environment. Organic germanium carries oxygen across cellular membranes into the cell, and helps fight diseases caused by insufficient cellular oxygenation. One study concluded that organic germanium restored the function of T-cells and B-lymphocytes (support immunity), and increased the number of antibody-forming cells, with no side effects.

Research indicates germanium might help treat cancer of the lungs, bladder, larynx, and breast, as well as leukemia, cirrhosis of the liver, depression, asthma, arthritis, heavy metal poisoning, sinus infections, diabetes, hypertension, and heart disease. Because of the significant effects of germanium on cancer cells, it might prove to be an invaluable benefit to cancer patients.

HONOKIOL

Honokiol, or Magnolia Bark Extract, is a powerful anticancer compound that comes from the bark of the Magnolia Officinalis tree. An ancient staple of Chinese medicine, honokiol safely offers a variety of long-term health benefits.

Pure honokiol works on a cellular level to stop cancer growth and disable the metastatic process. It also works against inflammation (major cause of cancer and disease) and infections, and is an antioxidant with one thousand times more potency than vitamin C. Honokiol also has anti-anxiety properties and helps relieve stress, a key factor in the inflammatory process of cancer.

When compared to a pharmaceutical drug such as diazepam (Valium), honokiol appears to be just as effective in its anti-anxiety activity, but without the strong sedative and addictive effects; it doesn't cause drowsiness or fatigue.

OTHER STUDIES HAVE SHOWN THAT HONOKIOL HELPS SUPPORT NORMAL BRAIN FUNCTION AND PROTECT THE BRAIN FROM ALZHEIMER'S DISEASE:

- Modulates brain activity and enzymes
- Increases "choline acetyltransferase" (transfer enzyme that helps synthesize neurotransmitters in brain) activity

- Inhibits "acetylcholinesterase" (neurotransmitter that stops muscle contraction)
- Stimulates acetylcholine release

POWERFUL ANTIOXIDANT PROTECTION:
Honokiol and magnolol (natural compound extracted from a particular magnolia bark tree, inhibit some metastatic cancers) are both strong antioxidants and can help protect cardiovascular health. Taiwanese researchers found that magnolia extract is one thousand times more potent than vitamin E in arresting cell damage, a major contributor to heart disease.

A number of studies have shown that magnolia extract protected the cells' energy resource from free-radical damage in the liver, heart, and brain of laboratory animals. Over the last several years, hundreds of clinical trials have been assessing magnolia's effect in treating various kinds of cancer.

SEVERAL STUDIES HAVE TESTED MAGNOLIA EXTRACT ON HUMAN CANCER CELLS AND FOUND IT A POWERFUL ANGIOGENESIS INHIBITOR:

- Might be an effective drug for leukemia
- Slows growth of human lung "squamous" carcinoma and other tumors
- Decreases cancer cells in human colon and liver tumors
- Enhances production of steroids by the adrenal cortex, which counteracts adrenal fatigue
- Inhibits bacteria and disease-causing fungi
- Reduces inflammation and pain
- Protects against seizures
- Antidote for pesticide poisoning
- Helps control and relieve asthma

No significant toxic or adverse effects have been reported to date when honokiol is taken as directed.

Scientists have also found that honokiol can help reduce the degenerative process of osteoporosis by improving bone growth and mineralization. It protects the body against the side effects of chemotherapy and radiation, and increases the benefits of other natural therapies, such as modified citrus pectin (MCP), which also has a variety of health benefits—more on that later.

STEM CELL TRANSPLANTS

Cancer Treatment Centers of America have aligned with an alternative, holistic medical model in their treatment of cancer. They provide advanced therapies for various stages of cancer, including leukemia, non-Hodgkin lymphoma, multiple myeloma, and other blood cancers. Some patients are given stem cell transplants for these particular cancers.

Stem cell transplants introduce healthy stem cells into the body to stimulate new bone marrow growth, suppress the cancer, and reduce the possibilities of relapse. This DNA renewal system stimulates growth factors and cytokines to facilitate stem cell production and activation.

A patient undergoes intensive, high doses of chemotherapy prior to the transplant to destroy as many cancer cells as possible. Then the patient is given stem cells intravenously. After an hour procedure, the stem cells travel to the bone marrow and make new healthy blood cells. These include red blood cells, which carry oxygen to the body; white blood cells, which help fight infections; and platelets, which control bleeding and clotting.

There are several types of transplants, depending on the nature of the disease. In *autotransplants*, the patient receives his own stem cells, which are taken and stored in a freezer until a course of chemotherapy is completed. In *allotransplants*, the patient receives stem cells from another person who is a donor match. And *umbilical cord transplants* are for patients who can't find a match, so cells are extracted from the umbilical cord of a baby.

Stem cell therapy is intended to cure diseases, and in many cases, patients have a 100 percent cure rate, while others are either in remission or the disease returns due to the body's inability to recover after conventional treatments, like chemotherapy and radiation. In some cases, stem cell therapy is ineffective due to the body's inability to accept the new cells.

In addition to the transplants, there are stem cell-enhancing supplements that support and nourish the immune system before and after treatment. Stemtech International is a company that provides supplements to support immunity, before and after transplants.

Stem cell therapy must be administered in a hospital or clinic, in a safe and clean environment. It's important the patient remain in a sterile environment also during chemotherapy treatment, due to the possibility of contracting outside pathogens.

It takes several months to recover from this procedure, and at the Cancer Treatment Centers of America, nutritionists and other specialists devise a personalized protocol to nourish the patient after treatment. They utilize natural therapies such as nutrition, herbs, and supplements to maximize the body's immune system. These specialists- nurses, doctors and holistic practitioners, help in the management of stress, visualization techniques, acupuncture, and discuss emotional and spiritual practices for optimum healing.

Stem cell therapy offers extraordinary promise not only in cancer treatments, but also in the treatment of paralysis, Alzheimer's, arthritis, and a host of other autoimmune disorders. Stem cells have extraordinary regenerative properties, revitalize cellular energy, and help improve the immune system, memory, skin, mood disorders, and muscle and bone strength.

AGS-GLYCOSIDE COMPONENT (ALGYCON SAPOGENIN)

AGS-Glycoside is a natural component and herbal extract of panax ginseng. It functions by bonding natural sugars in the body to a carbohydrate that separates them from each other; the carbohydrate becomes active, while the sugar becomes inactive, thereby deactivating the production of cancer cells. Since sugar feeds cancer, this process is effective in arresting sugar's ability to nourish cancer cells.

In 1999, a leading oncologist was sought out by a number of end-stage cancer patients who weren't responding to standard treatments. Because they were classified as terminal, the doctor gave them an innovative therapy that showed promise—a non-sugar component of a glycoside group called AGS.

The results were amazingly successful, and five years later 86 percent of those patients were still alive. Since then, this doctor has seen more successes with AGS, and his colleagues are dumbfounded by the results. Researchers have used AGS on melanoma tumors and reported noticeable results in as little as twenty-four hours.

AGS works by cutting off the blood supply (angiogenesis) of tumors without dissolving them chemically. Researchers also used AGS on cancer cells that had spread to patients' lungs, and it was reported that it reduced the lung tumors and stopped the spread of the disease almost immediately.

Just as germs become resistant to antibiotics, these new cancers become multiple-drug resistant. Doctors and scientists predict that within the next several years, at least four million people worldwide will soon die of these super-cancers. The numbers seem staggering, but considering the efficacy of many new cancer treatments and therapies, they might be significantly diminished in the coming decades.

Another asset of AGS is that it has no side effects. Tests of AGS have found that it's non-toxic and appears to be so non-invasive that people can take it regularly as a preventive measure.

Studies have shown that AGS works on colon, lung, ovarian, kidney, and brain cancers. Another physician from China, has even seen amazing results in patients with pancreatic cancer, the most volatile and deadly of cancers.

SEVERAL RESEARCH STUDIES OF AGS HAVE DISCOVERED THESE POWERFUL BENEFITS:

- Stimulates cell death (apoptosis) of tumors
- Kills cancers that are resistant to drugs
- Crosses the blood-brain barrier to kill brain cancer
- Does not affect healthy tissue
- Increases absorption of cancer drugs
- Eliminates toxins and excess estrogen (which might reduce incidences of hormone-receptive breast cancer)

Reports have stated that some patients have been cancer-free after only twenty-four hours after AGS treatment. Health professionals recommend AGS be given intravenously for the most effective results.

Pegasus Pharmaceuticals in Canada produces AGS in gel capsules. Another AGS product, Force C, is available without prescription.

ARTEMISININ

Dr. Henry Lai, Ph.D., bioengineering research professor at the University of Washington, has focused much of his research studying electromagnetic fields and their effects on biological tissue. One area of his research uses electromagnetic fields to treat diseases, such as destroying the malaria parasite through pulsing magnetic fields.

During a phone conversation in 1994, Dr. Lai asked a colleague who had just returned from a malaria seminar what was new in the field. His colleague told him, "Well, there is a new anti-malarial called artemisinin. Come over to my office and I'll give you a paper on it." Dr. Lai went over to his office, took the paper, and started reading it on his way back to his own office. Suddenly, the idea of using artemisinin to selectively kill cancer cells "jumped into my mind," he says. Dr. Lai had made the simple but profound connection to the known fact that all cancer cells sequester iron, just as the malaria parasite does.

In order to sequester iron needed for their rapid cell division, cancer cells have higher percentages of receptors that transport iron (called transferrin receptors) into the cells.

Breast cancer cells have five to fifteen times as many of these iron receptors as normal breast cells, and an elevated level of iron is a common finding in breast cancer tissue as well as in other cancer cells. Leukemia cells have the highest concentration of iron, up to one thousand times more iron than normal cells. This indicates that the iron is captured, or sequestered when cancer exists in the body, and can't be utilized to support blood in a healthy manner.

The breast cancer cell research resulted in a 28 percent reduction of breast cancer cells treated only with artemisinin, and a staggering 98 percent decrease in breast cancer cells that were treated with artemisinin and an iron-enhancing bioavailable molecule, transferrin, within sixteen hours after treatment. This is a significantly fast result.

These same treatments had no significant effect on normal human breast cells. This research pointed to the involvement of free iron in the toxic effect of artemisinin toward cancer cells, while basically sparing healthy cells. In other words, "free iron" supports artemisinin's ability to have a toxic effect on cancer cells, disabling them from metastasizing. These results become even more potentially important because the breast cancer cells used in the study were radiation-resistant, a difficult situation to overcome.

An earlier study of artemisinin with human leukemia cells demonstrated 100 percent cancer cell destruction in half the time (eight hours) than that of the breast cancer cells, probably due to the rapid cell division and higher iron concentration of leukemia cells. These results were encouraging, but often test-tube results do not carry over into animal testing, which was the next step.

Rats implanted with cancer (fibrosarcoma) and given iron (ferrous sulfate) followed by a form of artemisinin (dihydroartemisinin) had a significant reduction in the growth rate of the implanted tumors. There appeared to be no tumor growth reduction in rats given either substance, iron or artemisinin, alone.

Normally, at this point in research, the animal studies would be continued for several years with toxicity studies, and further studies proving the efficacy of the protocol. Then small human studies would start, again determining the toxicity levels and efficacy. This whole process takes years to complete before the general public has access to a new treatment.

The development of this treatment was different this time due to the fact that artemisinin and its derivatives have been available and in use for thirty years, and therefore are considered safe and non-toxic. The herb has been used by the Chinese for many centuries. Dr. Lai simply recognized a new use—cancer reduction, for an old substance.

Once physicians realized they didn't have to give their patients iron to make artemisinin potent in certain types of cancer, several started their terminal cancer patients on low doses. As word traveled through the cancer treatment network, many patients, who had exhausted all other options, also initiated self-treatment with artemisinin.

Several patients have called to report their successes to the Washington researchers. Although all the following stories must be considered anecdotal because they have not been part of a clinical, controlled study, they are exciting and hopeful for everyone who is dealing with the challenges of cancer.

Several cases of significant improvement of prostate cancer have been reported. One Belgian man, who started out with a PSA of 12, dropped his PSA down to under .38 within a short time.

Another man with a PSA of 4 dropped it down to 2 in six weeks. He was then feeling so well he went on a trip to South America and rode on a bicycle again. Another man lowered his PSA from

7.8 to 1.9 in three weeks. A doctor lowered his PSA from 3 down to .45 in six weeks.

A Canadian man with a pancreatic tumor and several liver tumors has been controlling his cancer for fifteen months with *artemisinin derivatives.*

Several stories of improvement in brain cancer have reached the researchers. One young boy with a glioblastoma in New York was confined to bed and unable to walk, but got up and attended a sporting event within ten days of taking artemether (synthetic form of arteminisin). A patient from Denmark had lost his hearing due to a brain tumor, and regained it after a regimen of artemether. Another young boy has been doing well without surgery or radiation.

Two outstanding cases of breast cancer successes were written up in Dr. Robert Rowen's article, entitled "Chinese Herb Cures Cancer," in the May 2002 issue of *Second Opinion*. One was a 47-year-old woman with fourth-stage breast cancer with metastases to her spine, which caused significant pain and limping. Various alternative therapies gave her some symptomatic relief, but no change was registered on her CT scan until a course of artemisinin was instituted.

Dr. Rowen's article also mentioned his success with a newly diagnosed case of lymphoma, manifesting as an egg-sized tumor on the left side of a man's head, which spontaneously cleared up two weeks after a two-week course of artemisinin derivatives.

To the scientific community, however, this might seem premature, but people who have exhausted their options are trying derivatives or synthetics of artemisinin in increasing numbers.

So far, anecdotal reports Dr. Singh has received show these derivatives provide some degree of cancer growth control, and if not remission, at least stabilization in every type of cancer tried.

The parent plant that the active compound comes from is called artemesia annua L.

Several semi-synthetic derivatives of artemisinin have been developed in efforts to increase absorption and stability, and reduce toxicity. Although several other derivatives are available, only the three forms that are presently being used by physicians will be discussed here—artemisinin, artesunate, and artemether.

All three of the forms are broken down at various rates in the body into several metabolites, the principle one being dihydroartemisinin (DHA). All three forms are absorbed fairly quickly after oral intake, but each reaches a peak concentration and has effects that last different lengths of time. All three forms go through the blood-brain barrier to some degree, but the fat-soluble form has superior absorption into the brain.

Artemisinin is the active natural extract from the herb. It is not at all water-soluble and has poorer absorption than some other forms. Artesunate, on the other hand, is quickly absorbed and reaches its peak concentration in the blood within forty minutes. This form is broken down very quickly into its metabolites in the liver, and excreted somewhat quickly, but still has some metabolic effects for as long as four hours.

Artemisinin is often given in a suppository form to children with malaria, extending its activity before it's metabolized, although rectal absorption of this compound is still somewhat limited.

A 500 mg capsule that has only 5 percent to 10 percent activity will only provide 25 mg to 50 mg of active compound, which might be too low to obtain any results. A 100 mg capsule with 100 percent activity is far more effective.

Artesunate is a semi-synthetic form that is more water-soluble. This form tends to break down easily when stored in hot climates, which is certainly a consideration for treating malaria. All the artemisinin compounds are light-sensitive, decomposing when exposed to light.

One study reported the absorption of artesunate is about 61 percent, and has the shortest activity period in the body, of the three forms. Some sources claim artesunate is the most active form, but this has not been proven.

Artemether is a semi-synthetic, more fat-soluble form that is the longest lasting in the bloodstream. Due to the fat-soluble nature of this compound, it passes more readily through the blood-brain barrier. It is also metabolized fairly rapidly to DHA, and blood tests show that after six hours, the DHA metabolite has higher plasma concentrations than the parent compound artemether.

HYPERTHERMIA

Deep-tissue hyperthermia is the use of heat, sometimes in combination with radiation therapy or chemotherapy, to treat certain cancers in the body. When cells in the body are exposed to higher than normal temperatures, changes take place inside the cells. These changes can make the cells more receptive to radiation therapy or chemotherapy treatment, both of which may be optional.

Deep-tissue hyperthermia is used to reach tumors located more than three centimeters under the skin surface, which includes most cancers. Prior to the procedure, a CT scan is performed to precisely locate the tumor area. Then temperature probes accurately monitor external and internal temperatures.

A water-filled applicator is then placed over the patient's abdomen, and focused electromagnetic energy (radio frequency energy) is directed at the tumor, heating the tumor to a temperature between 104 degrees to 107 degrees Fahrenheit. Deep-tissue hyperthermia dilates blood vessels around the tumor, causing oxygen-carrying red blood cells to spread into the tumor. Oxygen floods the tumor cells, and the cancer literally suffocates and dies.

If the patient is later exposed to radiation treatment, the radiation reacts with the high levels of oxygen in the tumor, potentially destroying the cancer cells. If the patient receives chemotherapy, the increased blood flow to the tumor area might bring more chemotherapy to the tumor. Cancer cells can be weakened or destroyed, while healthy tissue is typically not damaged.

Research shows that high temperatures can damage and kill cancer cells, usually with minimal injury to normal tissues. It's indicated that by killing cancer cells and damaging proteins and structures within the cells, hyperthermia treatment might shrink tumors, according to the National Cancer Institute. Preliminary data suggest heat might be especially destructive to two types of tumor cells—those making deoxyribonucleic acid (DNA) in preparation for division, and those that are acidic and poorly oxygenated. These cell types tend to be resistant to radiation.

Whole body hyperthermia (WBH) treatment, achieved with either radiant heat or extracorporeal technologies, increases the temperature of the entire body to at least 41 degrees Celsius. In radiant WBH, heat is externally applied to the whole body using hot-water blankets, hot wax, inductive coils, or thermal chambers. The patient is sedated throughout the WBH procedure, which lasts approximately four hours. The patient reaches target temperature within approximately 1.3 hours, is maintained at 41.8 degrees Celsius for one hour, and experiences a one-hour cooling phase.

During treatment, the esophageal, rectal, skin, and ambient air temperatures are monitored at ten-minute intervals. Small probes may be inserted into the tumor under a local anesthetic to monitor the temperature of the affected and surrounding tissue. Heart rate, respiratory rate, and cardiac rhythm are continuously monitored. Patients are returned to regular in-patient rooms after hyperthermia cancer treatment and discharged after twenty to twenty-four hours of observation.

Extracorporeal WBH is achieved by reinfusion of extracorporeally heated blood. A circuit of blood is created outside the body by accessing an artery, usually the femoral artery, and creating an extracorporeal loop. The circulating blood is passed through a heating device, often a water bath or hot air, and the heated blood is then reinjected into a major vein. The desired body temperature is adjusted and controlled by changing the volume flow of the warmed reinfused blood. Extracorporeal hyperthermia treatments are conducted under general anesthesia.

To counteract the activation of coagulation by the blood infuser, high-dose heparin is sometimes administered to prevent blood clots. Target temperature is reached in two hours and is maintained for one hour, followed by a cooling period of one hour.

Afterwards, the patient is infused with normal saline to maintain systolic blood pressure above 100 mm Hg. The patient is then monitored weekly for possible complications.

This treatment is another example of the revolutionary alternative protocols for cancer, and how they affect the whole body without causing damage to healthy cells and tissues.

NALTREXONE

Naltrexone is a pharmaceutical drug that works by activating the body's immune system against disease. It targets the growth factor in some cancers and blocks the rapid reproduction of cancer cells. Naltrexone works with brain-based endorphins, which interact with the immune system, pain, and the growth of blood vessels that feed a tumor (angiogenesis). In other words, Naltrexone works to reduce the proliferation of cancerous cells by increasing endorphins in the brain.

In addition, this drug also has a potent effect on other autoimmune disorders, such as irritable bowel syndrome (IBS), Crohn's, autism, lupus, chronic fatigue, HIV virus, and hepatitis C.

Side effects might be similar to chemotherapy, and Naltrexone is not considered a natural therapy. It's thought to be safe, however, and effectively treats cancer, in many cases.

All of these diseases, as well as cancer, are related to low levels of endorphins in the body. Low blood levels of endorphins contribute to all immune deficiencies. Several studies have been conducted on Naltrexone, and the results show promise in treating lung, liver, breast, ovarian, lymphatic, colon, and rectal cancers.

Naltrexone has been approved by the FDA for over twenty years, often used to treat alcohol and drug addictions, but because the doses in treating these cancers are so low, it's not profitable for pharmaceutical companies to support it. *As a result, few doctors are aware of the effectiveness of this substance, and clinical trials have been limited.*

A few compounding pharmacies in the United States and Canada distribute Naltrexone for professional use.

METFORMIN

Metformin is a compound traditionally used to treat diabetes, but clinical trials are investigating its potential in preventing specific cancers such as endometrial, colon, prostate, and breast cancers. The effectiveness of Metformin is related to its function, which is to control blood sugar levels and thereby control the sugar intake of cancer cells (sugar feeds cancer cells). Studies indicate that Metformin induces apoptosis (the death of cancer cells) in early stages of development through the same pathways that promote weight loss, by regulating how sugar is processed in the body.

Control study groups have found that patients prescribed Metformin along with traditional treatments, appeared to have a higher success rate in reducing tumors and their reproduction. Studies also show that patients given the drug preventatively were much less likely to develop cancer than those who didn't take the drug.

Due to these findings, scientists have begun several clinical trials to determine the effect of Metformin on breast and other cancers. Although it's a relatively recent finding, the possibilities of utilizing this compound in cancer treatment are highly promising, and offer a greatly effective alternative to traditional invasive medicine.

CYTOKINE THERAPY

Cytokines, which are intercellular proteins known to play a role in maintaining and regulating immunity and inflammatory processes, are a natural alternative for the control of diseases, including cancer. The extensive use of antibiotics and chemicals in animals has resulted in environmental and human health concerns, believed to contribute to the increase in cancer and autoimmune diseases.

The World Health Organization has urged meat producers to use environmentally friendly methods to reduce antibiotics and toxins in our foods. Unfortunately, some producers genetically modify foods using seeds and pesticides that affect organ function in animals and humans. This practice has increased the number of cancer-causing agents exponentially, and therefore, the need for effective natural treatments is now more significant than ever.

Cytokines, natural regulators of the immune system, offer effective alternatives to conventional therapies. They are familiar substances, such as interleuken, interferon and other proteins, that are secreted by the cells and have a regenerative effect on the immune system. They help cell communication, regulate pain, inflammation, and blood cell development and formation, functioning similarly to stem cell therapy.

The use of cytokines has become even more feasible with the recent cloning of a number of cytokine genes. Since the chicken's immune system is similar to that of humans, it offers an appropriate method with which to study the effectiveness of cytokine therapy in the control of disease.

Cytokine therapy has proven to help treat patients with advanced cancer. This therapy manipulates the immune response to generate the appropriate immune-potent cells for eliminating tumors. It has been administered with positive results to tumors in patients with renal cancer and melanoma.

The negative aspect of this therapy is that cytokines can create a level of toxicity, as do chemotherapy and radiation. As with chemo, common toxicities cause nausea, vomiting, fever, chills, fatigue, and headaches. Therefore, it's necessary to carefully monitor levels of cytokines to avoid harming the cells or blood.

Researchers found that one type of cytokine, called "multiferon," can enhance a patient's immune response to cancer cells by activating certain white blood cells, such as natural killer cells and T-cells. Multiferon might also impede the growth of cancer cells and promote their death. This particular cytokine is approved for the treatment of melanoma, Kaposi's sarcoma, and several other blood cancers.

"Hematopoietic" stem cells are blood cells that create all other blood cells and are located in the bone marrow. All blood cells originate from these stem cells in the bone marrow. Because chemotherapy drugs target growing blood cells, including normal stem cells, chemotherapy depletes these stem cells and the blood cells they produce. Loss of red blood cells, which transport oxygen and nutrients throughout the body, can cause anemia. A decrease in platelets, which maintain blood clotting, might lead to profuse bleeding. Cytokines enable the body to fight natural killer cells by enhancing immunity.

Several growth factors that promote the production of these various blood cell populations are approved for clinical use. They are a significant benefit to the use of cytokines in cancer treatment:

- Erythropoietin stimulates the formation of red blood cells, and Interleukin 11 (IL-11) increases platelet production.
- Granulocyte-macrophage colony stimulating factor (GM-CSF) and granulocyte colony-stimulating factor (G-CSF) both increase the number of white blood cells, reducing the risk of infections. G-CSF and GM-CSF can enhance the immune system's anticancer responses by increasing the number of T-cells.

Treatment with cytokines may prove to make a significant contribution to the treatment of specific cancers, and more research is necessary.

FUCOIDAN

Fucoidan is a sulfated polysaccharide extracted from brown seaweed, thought to be involved in the stem cell-induced repair of heart disease, cancer, and other pathogenic illness. The Chinese refer to Fucoidan as "virgin mother's milk" because it contains the same nutrients and healing properties as breast milk.

FUCOIDAN HEALTH BENEFITS:

- Anti-cancer
- Immunity builder
- Anti-inflammatory
- Stem cell regenerator

Researchers have stated that Fucoidan has more valuable and anti-cancer agents than any one substance.

These are factors to consider when searching for the appropriate Fucoidan supplement:

- A source free of radiation (oceans have high levels of radiation from Fukushima, and other toxic chemicals)
- Bioavailability and containing proper amounts of marine molecules
- Effective dose for therapeutic use

Eight Essential Saccharides (Sugars) That Add To Fucoidan Health Benefits and Enhance Cellular Communication:

1. Mannose

- Prevents bacterial, viral, parasitic, and fungal infections
- Eases inflammation
- This saccharide is particularly indicated for lupus patients
- Lowers blood sugar and triglyceride levels in diabetic patients

2. Fucose

- Increases growth factors identical to those found in breast milk
- Influences brain development and long-term memory
- Induces production of interferon and interleukin
- Regulates the immune system
- Activates stem cells
- Creates longevity factors
- Inhibits tumor growth through apoptosis
- Active against herpes simplex 1 and other viruses associated with chickenpox
- Guards against respiratory infections
- Inhibits allergic reactions by suppressing allergy associated antibodies

- Increases growth factors for muscle rebuilding
- Stimulates bone growth and repair
- Creates growth factors for skin, hair, lining of internal organs
- Anti-inflammatory
- Re-pigments graying hair
- Increases energy
- Protects eyes and major organs

3. Galactose

- Enhances wound healing
- Increases calcium absorption
- Helps long-term memory

4. Glucose

- Powerful fast-energy source
- Enhances memory
- Stimulates calcium absorption

Elderly Alzheimer's patients register lower levels of healthy glucose than those with organic brain disease from stroke or other vascular diseases.

- Glucose metabolism disturbed in depression, manic-depression, anorexia, and bulimia

5. N-Acetylgalactosamine

- In low levels, might cause susceptibility to heart disease
- Inhibits spread of tumor
- Immune modulator with anti-cancer properties
- Activity against HIV

6. N-Acetylglucosamine

- Vital to cognitive activity
- Glucosamine is a metabolic product of this
- Helps repair cartilage
- Decreases pain and inflammation
- Increases range of movement
- Repairs lining of gut in Crohn's disease, ulcerative colitis, and cystitis

7. N-Acetylneuraminic Acid

- Stimulates brain development and learning
- Repels bacteria, virus, and fungi
- Abundant in breast milk

8. Xylose

- Antibacterial and antifungal
- Known to prevent cancer of the digestive tract

Fucoidan is scientifically proven to cause cancer cells to self-destruct.

GERSON THERAPY

Gerson Therapy is a natural treatment that supports the body's own ability to heal. This is accomplished through an organic raw-juice diet, natural supplements and herbs, and coffee enemas. This plant-based diet boosts the immune system to detoxify and heal autoimmune, inflammatory, and degenerative diseases, including cancer.

There is a significant amount of available information on the efficacy of Gerson Therapy, and numerous testimonials from people who've been "cured" from cancer and other autoimmune disorders. There are patients who have spent a week at the clinic with significant improvements or are "cured," and others who have spent weeks or months using the Gerson protocol and have returned home in remission and asymptomatic. There are, of course, always less successful stories, but the majority of patients who have returned home are significantly healthier than before they arrived.

The success of the treatment depends on the nature, degree and progression of the cancer, and also on the holistic health of the patient. The clinic offers group therapy sessions, along with yoga practices and other kinds of spiritual and visualization participation to give the patient an overall approach to healing.

The premise of the treatment is that inflammation and toxicity cause illness, especially cancer. Gerson Therapy provides a safe, natural detoxification process and diet, enhancing immunity, reducing inflammation, and stimulating the regeneration of healthy cells. The Gerson Institute is located in Mexico.

VIRAL INFUSIONS

Scientists and researchers are now using specific viruses as therapy for the treatment of cancer. They have discovered that certain viruses, in a modified state when injected into tumors, miraculously eliminate cancer cells in some patients. More research and evaluation are currently being conducted, but this therapy might prove to be on the cutting edge of science in the treatment of cancer.

ELECTRO-MAGNETIC PULSE AND INFUSIONS

Electro-magnetic pulse (EMP) machines and instruments, such as the Zapper, stimulate the body's own healing processes. The

Zapper, which sends electro-magnetic pulsations throughout the body or into specific areas, is known to zap out pathogens, chemicals, and other toxins, including parasites. EMP machines are also known to significantly increase the potency of other treatments and infusions, when used simultaneously. They boost healthy immune cells, suppress tumor growth, reduce inflammation and pain, and stimulate detoxification.

CUTTING EDGE

Massive doses of vitamin and mineral therapies, particularly vitamin C, are also known to starve cancer cells by flooding the body with antioxidants, thereby oxygenating the cells. EMP and these intravenous therapies work synergistically to energize antioxidants in the body to fight off pathogens, such as cancer.

The treatments and therapies outlined in this book are only a few of the more than one hundred protocols for treating cancer. Research to discover alternative natural therapies are constantly in motion, and new developments appear on a regular basis. We are very fortunate to be at the forefront of possible cures for a variety of diseases, cancer being the most devastating and invasive of all.

This is a call to action to implore the scientific and medical communities to continue to do research, expand, explore and experiment on natural, alternative therapies for cancer. This is a momentous time in our history, and only a glimpse of what we can expect in the future.

CHAPTER 6

AUTOIMMUNE DISORDERS, SYMPTOMS AND TREATMENTS

Autoimmunity is a factor in more than one hundred diseases, disorders, and syndromes. Many people suffer from them unknowingly, and some with no solution in sight. This information is intended to shed light on these problems: to discuss what autoimmune diseases are, how they are identified, and to suggest solutions. Autoimmune disorders have increased rapidly in modern society, and it's imperative that we utilize the increasing numbers of available treatments.

TREATING AUTOIMMUNE DISORDERS

Although they manifest in different ways, feel different, look different, and might be evaluated and treated differently, all of these disorders originate from a weakened immune system caused by chemical toxins, candida, inflammation, virus, bacteria, parasites and other pathogens.

Autoimmune disorders are evaluated using a variety of different kinds of tests, both medical and holistic, which usually determine the nature of the disease. If not given the appropriate attention or treatments, they might eventually lead to extreme pathology, debilitation, depression, exhaustion, and in some cases, fatality.

This guide is crucially important for those of you who are desperate to find answers, and locate a practitioner who understands your suffering and doesn't tell you it's "all in your head."

GENERAL SYMPTOMS OF AUTOIMMUNE DISORDERS:

If you identify with more than eight to ten of the following symptoms, chances are it's time to visit an autoimmune specialist, immunologist, or other qualified professional, who can evaluate the problem and help guide you toward solutions.

EXTREME FATIGUE—daily exhaustion that rest or sleep doesn't remedy, experienced almost across the board by autoimmune patients

MUSCLE AND JOINT PAIN—pain, burning, aches, and soreness in muscles and joint, present in most autoimmune disorders

MUSCLE WEAKNESS—weak muscles and lack of strength in limbs

SWOLLEN GLANDS—anywhere in the body, especially around the throat, underarms, tops of legs, and groin area

INFLAMMATION—present generally or specifically in the body with all autoimmune disorders

SUSCEPTIBILITY TO INFECTIONS—frequent colds, sore throats, and bladder, ear, sinus, and yeast infections, with slower recovery periods

SLEEP DISTURBANCES—difficulty falling asleep and/or frequent waking

WEIGHT LOSS OR GAIN—changes in weight more distinct than usual

LOW BLOOD SUGAR—adrenal fatigue, fluctuations in insulin, and anemia

BLOOD PRESSURE CHANGES—low blood pressure due to fatigue, or high blood pressure with dizziness, fainting spells, heart palpitations, and fluctuations in heart rate

CANDIDA YEAST INFECTIONS—related to digestive problems, sinus infections, gas bloating, vaginal yeast, mouth thrush, depression, irritability, mood changes, muscle or joint pain, rashes, mental confusion, disorientation, and more

ALLERGIES—sensitivities to foods, mold, chemicals, and toxins

DIGESTIVE PROBLEMS—can include abdominal pain, bloating, tenderness, heartburn, cramps, constipation, diarrhea, gas, and leaky gut syndrome

ANXIETY AND DEPRESSION—can include mood and emotional swings, panic attacks, excessive irritability, and irrationality

MEMORY PROBLEMS—can include brain fog, confusion, and memory loss

THYROID PROBLEMS—hypothyroidism (low thyroid), hyperthyroidism, low body temperature, and excessive hair loss

HEADACHES—migraines as well as recurring or dull headaches

LOW-GRADE FEVERS—a common occurrence with auto-immune deficiencies, as the body works harder to stave off infections

PREMENTRUAL SYNDROME—increase in typical PMS symptoms, extreme bloating, cramps, heavy bleeding, and menstrual irregularity

MISCARRIAGE—spontaneous miscarriage might indicate immune deficiency

INTRODUCTION TO AUTOIMMUNE DISORDERS

Always confer with your health care practitioner before any treatment, since circumstances sometimes indicate a different approach is necessary.

In addition, it's important to note that not all symptoms accompany any or all of these disorders; they vary according to the person and level of illness. The same applies to treatment, which is based on individual needs and requirements, strictly in accordance with your practitioner's recommendations. What is effective for some may not be effective for all, which is another significant factor in the outcome of any healing program. These are strictly suggestions and recommendations for treatment.

AUTOIMMUNE DISORDERS AND RECOMMENDED TREATMENTS

ALZHEIMER'S DISEASE

SYMPTOMS Memory problems, confusion, disorientation, mood swings, depression, dementia, inability to handle simple tasks, inappropriate behavior, episodes of violence or rage

TREATMENTS Vitamins A, C, D, E, and B complex; turmeric; fiber; fish oils; no processed or junk foods; choline chloride; L-carnitine; DHA; ginkgo biloba; caprylic acid; coconut oil; CoQ10; glutathione; chelation therapy; phosphatidylserine for detoxification of heavy metals in the brain

AMYOTROPHIC LATERAL SCLEROSIS (ALS)

SYMPTOMS Muscle weakness in hands and limbs, impaired speech, twitching, shortness of breath, paralysis, loss of bodily functions

TREATMENT Detoxification of heavy metals and chemical toxins from the brain, liver, and intestines; candida cleanse; balancing of sulfur and selenium levels; high omega 3-6-9 fatty acid doses; large doses of multivitamins and minerals; creatinine; turmeric; dandelion; cinnamon; colloidal gold; cayenne; goldenseal root; coconut oil to revive dead neurons in the brain; mega green leafy vegetables; healthful diet; physical therapy.

ANEMIA

SYMPTOMS Fatigue, muscle weakness, headaches, dizziness, fainting, heart palpitations, shortness of breath, pale skin and lips, cold hands and feet, menstrual weakness

TREATMENT Iron, green leafy vegetables; blackstrap molasses, pumpkin seeds, beetroot, chlorophyll; dong quai (Chinese herb that builds blood), Oregon grape; Asian ginseng; parsley, nettle, goldenseal, hawthorn berry, gentian, alfalfa, watercress; brewer's yeast, vitamins C and B12; folic acid, spirulina, yellow dock

ARTHRITIS

SYMPTOMS Inflammation, stiffness and pain in joints, deformity of joints, fatigue, weakness, swelling, discomfort moving, restricted range of motion

TREAMENT Overall detoxification; aloe vera liquid; mustard seed, olive oil, cedarwood oil and myrrh (topically); omegas 3-6-9; fiber, green vegetables, low-acid foods; raw pineapple, bromelain for inflammation; MSM; high-potency multivitamin betaine HCL, cayenne, turmeric, ginger, garlic, boswellia for inflammation

CANCER

SYMPTOMS Unexplained weight loss; bone pain; persistent low-grade fever; recurrent infections; persistent cough or cough with blood; swollen lymph glands; bloating; changes in breasts; anemia; persistent fatigue, nausea, or vomiting; mole or wart that changes shape, color, or thickness; sore that heals slowly; lump or swelling under the skin; difficulty swallowing; change in bowels or bleeding; recurring headaches

TREATMENT Detoxification, clean balanced diet; alkaline foods, lots of green vegetables, fiber, olive oil, primrose, black seed and black currant oils; green tea, seaweed, vitamins A and B; mega-doses of intravenous vitamins C and E; beta-carotene, selenium, cesium chloride, turmeric, proteolytic enzymes (takes off protein coating of cancer cells so immune system recognizes unnatural cells); glutathione, CoQ10, grape-seed extract, DHEA, enzymes, zinc, chromium, astragalus, garlic, echinacea, ginger, turmeric, ginseng; oxygen treatments; medical ozone therapy

CANDIDIASIS OR CANDIDA

SYMPTOMS Low energy, irritability, anxiety, fear, depression, brain fog, memory loss, headaches, muscle and joint pain; sensitivity to chemicals; allergies, infections, vaginal itching and discharge; heart palpitations, sinusitis and respiratory problems; eczema, acne, diarrhea, stomach cramps, sugar cravings; general debilitation

TREATMENT Detoxification, candida cleansing diet, and supplements are key elements; fatty acids; vitamins C and B complex; chlorophyll; garlic; black walnut tincture; Pau d'Arco; Oregon grape and chamomile; Candida Cleanse or other products; grapefruit seed, olive leaf, and oregano oil extracts; colloidal silver; peppermint; milk thistle, caprylic acid; gentian root; high-potency probiotic supplements (see Candida chapter)

CHRONIC FATIGUE SYNDROME (EPSTEIN-BARR VIRUS)

SYMPTOMS Weakness, exhaustion, loss of appetite, nausea, night sweats, allergies, chills; respiratory infections, sore throat, intestinal problems; sore or swollen lymph glands; low-grade fever, headaches, sleep disturbances; depression, anxiety, difficulty concentrating, loss of memory; joint pain, breathing problems, brain fog

TREATMENTS Immune-building foods; no processed foods, caffeine, sugar, or foods that drain energy; B complex; magnesium; DHEA; CoQ10; vitamins A, C, E and D; bioflavonoids; iron; zinc; potassium; magnesium; iodine; tyrosine; phenylalanine; linoleic acid; flax and pumpkin seeds; saw palmetto; wild yam; passion flower; feverfew; chasteberry; mangosteen; D-limonene (digestion, detoxification); glutathione; NADH (complexes from vitamin B3) Coenzyme 1 to help build energy; probiotic; omega fatty acids 3-6-9; L-carnitine; ginseng; St. John's wort; 5-HTP; olive leaf extract; oregano oil; colloidal silver (antiviral); ashwagandha (calming agent); turmeric; ginger; mistletoe; scullcap; licorice root

CROHN'S DISEASE

SYMPTOMS Abdominal pain, chronic diarrhea, gas, loss of appetite; weight loss; inflammation, nausea, fatigue; depression, mouth and anal sores; headaches, low-grade fever; anemia

TREATMENT Fresh organic foods; no refined carbohydrates; aloe vera juice, DGL licorice; fish oil, digestive enzymes, glutamine, zinc, glutathione; acupuncture; probiotics, chamomile, peppermint; alfalfa, dandelion, propolis, goldenseal, echinacea, lemongrass, slippery elm; oregano, turmeric, cat's claw, boswellia (anti-inflammatory); omegas3-6-9, borage oil, black currant oil, chlorella; sublingual B12, folic acid; multivitamin spectrum; green tea, marshmallow

CHRONIC HEADACHES

SYMPTOMS Migraines are characterized by severe pain on one or both sides of head with sensitivity to light; dizziness, nausea, vomiting, visual impairment. **Cluster headaches** are severe headaches on one side of the head that last for a few days before disappearing. **Tension headaches** feel like there's a band around the head, with pressure or throbbing anywhere around the head, as well as tension in the neck or shoulders.

TREATMENTS Avoid food additives, dairy, processed foods, wheat and sugar; eat fiber; calcium; magnesium; riboflavin;

feverfew (herb for migraines); 5-HTP to help circulation in blood vessels; ginkgo; melatonin; peppermint, ginger, turmeric; black or green tea; valerian; dong quai; coriander, yarrow, hops, mullein, rosemary; menthol; white willow bark (aspirin); digestive enzymes, probiotics

HERPES

SYMPTOMS Burning, tingling sensations, red blisters, cluster blisters; itching, throbbing pain; flu-like symptoms, fever, chills, swollen glands and lymph nodes; pain in throat; headaches

TREATMENT Avoid acidic foods, caffeine, sugar and L-arginine; take lysine; flaxseed, fish oil; H-Plex Defense (powerful supplement with vitamins and herbs); lemon balm extract, peppermint; prunella, sage, thyme, rosemary, chamomile; olive leaf extract; cayenne; astragalus; lomatium root (antiviral properties); oregano oil, colloidal silve, isatis root; propolis ointment; vitamin C; zinc topically or internally; licorice root; B-complex; probiotics; echinacea, multivitamins; super green foods, raw thymus

HYPOTHYROIDISM (UNDERACTIVE THYROID)

SYMPTOMS Fatigue, depression, irritability, weight gain; muscle aches; sensitivity to cold and heat; constipation; recurring infections; high cholesterol, hair loss, dry skin; insomnia, infertility, anxiety, low libido; memory loss; lowered immunity, water retention, anemia; tingling of hands and feet

TREATMENT Reduce sugar intake, caffeine, refined carbohydrates, and gluten; eat iodine rich foods; omega fatty acids; glutathione, glutamine, milk thistle, turmeric, chlorella, cilantro to detoxify heavy metals; flaxseed, coconut oil, apple cider vinegar;

fish; walnuts; mineral and amino acid complex; vitamins A and D; selenium, zinc; fiber; thyroid glandular, pituitary glandular, L-tyrosine (synthesizes thyroid hormone)

The use of glutamine is controversial. It's contraindicated for several conditions, so check in with your professional before usage.

ENVIRONMENTAL ILLNESS

SYMPTOMS Extreme fatigue; muscle aches, allergies, asthma, flu-like symptoms; ringing in the ears; heart palpitations; intestinal and digestive problems; sleep problems; loss of balance; skin disorders; memory loss, anxiety or panic, depression; sensitivities to hot and cold; manifestation of other autoimmune disorders (difficult to diagnose and treat by Western medical model)

TREATMENT Detoxification of liver, kidneys, and colon; clean diet with no refined foods, sugar, or caffeine; powerful antioxidant vitamins; glutamine, glutathione, L-carnitine, magnesium, folic acid, iron, zinc, selenium; probiotics; spirulina; thymus extract to stimulate immunity; glucosamine; black seed, chlorophyll, manganese; chelation therapy to rid the body of heavy metals

FIBROMYALGIA

SYMPTOMS Unexplained and widespread pain; pain in major trigger points (evaluated by practitioner); fatigue, anxiety; tingling sensations; depression, irritability; sensitivity to noise, light, and weather; joint pain; headache

TREATMENT Detoxification; lymphatic massage; acupuncture; healthful green superfoods; high-potency vitamins C, D, E, A, and B's, including B12; omega-3-6-9; magnesium, selenium, zinc, kelp, malic acid; 5-HTP; MSM for pain and inflammation; SAMe (improves mood); CoQ10; milk thistle; alpha lipoic acid; grape seed; nicotinamide adenine dinucleotide (NADH); valerian to calm nerves, passion flower, ashwagandha, hops

INSOMNIA
SYMPTOMS Inability to fall asleep, stay asleep, or both

TREATMENT Avoid alcohol, caffeine, sugar, and chocolate; eat foods high in tryptophan, like turkey; calcium, magnesium; B-complex; 5-HTP, melatonin, passion flower, magnolia bark, ashwagandha, chamomile, valerian, hops, chamomile, wild lettuce, California poppy, lemon balm, St. John's wort, B12

IRRITABLE BOWEL SYNDROME
SYMPTOMS Constipation, diarrhea; mucus or blood in stools; abdominal pain, inflammation, gas, nausea, headache; fatigue; intolerance to spicy foods and roughage; rumbling in stomach; belching, heartburn, occasional vomiting; bad taste in mouth; bloating; depression, anxiety, mental fog, insomnia

TREATMENT Detoxification; soluble-fiber diet; cooked vegetables; probiotics; peppermint oil; gentian root; acacia powder; fennel; digestive enzymes, ginger root, skullcap, aloe juice, slippery elm, artichoke leaf extract; glutamine, glutathione, betaine hydrochloride; avoid salads, roughage, caffeine, sugar, chocolate, oranges, and acidic foods

LUPUS
SYMPTOMS Recurring bladder infections and kidney problems; butterfly-shaped facial rash; fever, fatigue, weakness; joint and

muscle pain; weight loss, hair loss, sensitivity to sun; mouth sores; recurring infections; swelling in lymph nodes; nausea, constipation or diarrhea

TREATMENT Detoxification; foods high in sulfur for cartilage damage; healthful greens; protein-rich diet; fish oils, plant sterols to balance immune system; DHEA; B6; hydrochloric acid; omega fatty acids; borage oil; gentian root; MSM; digestive enzymes, boswellia, turmeric, multivitamins; probiotics; green tea; evening primrose, milk thistle, ginkgo biloba for circulation in kidneys, devil's claw, ginger, garlic, white willow bark and capsicum for pain relief; burdock, ashwagandha, echinacea, feverfew, goldenseal, Pau d'Arco

LYME DISEASE

SYMPTOMS Bull's-eye inflamed rash on leg; fevers, chills, rash, weight loss or gain; fatigue; twitching; flu-like symptoms; headaches, neck aches; tingling, facial paralysis; mood swings, panic attacks, irritability, depression

TREATMENT Detoxification, glutathione; andrographis (natural antibiotic); resveratrol, turmeric, cat's claw, glutamine; fruits and vegetables; nuts and seeds; intravenous vitamins such as A, D C, B, B6, and B12; chromium, magnesium, zinc, manganese, copper, molybdenum, selenium; probiotics; green tea; organic germanium to stimulate immune function; kelp, echinacea, goldenseal, milk thistle, red clover to clean blood

MULTIPLE SCLEROSIS

SYMPTOMS Loss of balance; poor coordination; constipation; staggering gait; muscle tremors; bowel or bladder incontinence;

blindness; paralysis; extreme fatigue; blurred vision, dizziness, impaired speech; facial paralysis; numbness or weakness in limbs

TREATMENT Detoxification and candida cleanse; remove mercury from dental fillings; glutathione, glutamine, fish oils, B12, high-potency vitamins (extra D3); plant sterols; digestive enzymes; gamma linoleic acid (anti-inflammatory); E-complex, K2, alpha lipoic acid, turmeric, carnitine, flaxseed, garlic, L-cysteine, inositol, choline; CoQ10; niacin; ginkgo biloba, echinacea, ginseng, St. John's wort, ashwagandha, DHEA, super-greens; milk thistle, chlorella, spirulina

PARKINSON'S DISEASE

SYMPTOMS Stiff expression; drooling; heavy feeling in arms and legs; rigid muscles; impaired balance, tremors; constipation; difficulty speaking; shuffling gait, stooped posture; inability to perform voluntary movements

TREATMENT Detoxification; raw foods; heavy doses of antioxidants, high fiber, fresh vegetable juices; avoidance of foods that cause inflammation; CoQ10, omega-3-6-9, NADH; N-acetylcysteine, which increases levels of glutathione; lipoic acid; selenium, melatonin, pregnenolone (supports cognition, anti-inflammatory), turmeric, ginkgo biloba, milk thistle for detoxifying; green tea; calcium and magnesium; passion flower, skullcap, and valerian

PSORIASIS

SYMPTOMS Red, inflamed patches of skin; thick, dry skin; distorted nails; blisters anywhere on the body; itching; burning; pain

TREATMENT Detoxification; alkaline; anti-inflammatory and candida diet; fish; fiber, whole grains, beans; hydrochloric acid for digestion; fish oil; capsaicin; sarsaparilla to reduce toxins, milk thistle, vitamins B12, D3 and C; apple cider vinegar; super-green foods; digestive enzymes; flaxseed oil to reduce inflammation; reishi mushroom; probiotics; gentian root; turmeric, ginger, garlic, willow bar,; Oregon grape, aloe juice; topical baking soda paste, tea tree oil

PULMONARY FIBROSIS

SYMPTOMS Fibrous scarring in lungs, which causes shortness of breath; dry cough; fatigue; rounding of tips of fingers or toes; muscle and joint aches; weight loss

TREATMENT Tibetan Herbal Balance Lung Support; Neprinol AFD; HCP Formulas Fibrenza; N-acetylcysteine, serrapeptase and nattokinase (antioxidants); no dairy, sugar, wheat, or gluten; anti-inflammatory diet; turmeric, boswellia, cat's claw, garlic, ginger

SHINGLES

SYMPTOMS Shingles is a virus that lives in the nerves; pain or itching on one side of chest and back or face; fever, chills, flu-like symptoms; headache; clear blisters that turn yellow and fill with fluid or fall off

TREATMENT High doses of B vitamins; spirulina; brewer's yeast; whole grains; vegetables; vitamin C, D, and E, high doses of vitamin A; avoid acidic foods; drink unsweetened cranberry juice; alkaline foods; capsaicin cream; olive leaf extract, oregano oil, colloidal silver; vitamin E-complex; lomatium root for immune support, St. John's Wort; nettle, red clover, aloe, ginseng, cayenne pepper, peppermint, thyme, licorice root, cat's claw, zinc

SINUSITIS

SYMPTOMS Congested nasal passages; pain and swelling; toothache; fatigue, fever, chills, flu symptoms; irritability; most sinus infections are viral; antibiotics helpful only if bacterial infection

TREATMENT Detoxification; no dairy, sugar, caffeine, or inflammatory foods; garlic, cayenne, flaxseed; probiotics; echinacea, goldenseal, oregano oil; N-acetylcysteine; bromelain to reduce inflammation; grapefruit seed extract (natural antibiotic); colloidal silver, oregano oil, olive leaf extract, andrographis (if bacterial); vitamin C and other antioxidants; grape-seed extract, elderflower, garlic, ginger, cayenne, turmeric; saltwater nasal wash for sinus drainage

KEY TO GOOD HEALTH

Autoimmune disorders affect the entire body and need to be addressed holistically. Treating symptoms is not effective; unless you address the core of the problem, which usually lies in the gut and immune system, it's doubtful you can get the results you desire.

There are several other less common autoimmune disorders. They all, in one way or another, are caused by a compromised, weakened immune system which began at birth, or somewhere along the way.

Diet, environment, allergies, chemicals, supplements, vaccinations and medications all play a crucial role in these diseases. Unfortunately, medications are only palliative, not curative, and can cause damage to the organs and tissues.

The key to good health is balance—physically, emotionally, mentally, and spiritually. It's recommended that you be your own health advocate and get second or even third opinions if you aren't getting answers, and take a holistic approach to your own body.

CHAPTER 7

IMMUNE SUPPORT PROTOCOLS

These immune support protocols are effective and serve a variety of functions in healing illness and supporting the immune system. They have been implemented by both Western and alternative, integrative medical doctors, and by holistic practitioners. They are all, in some way, supportive to immunity, which means they are used both to prevent and treat disease. The results, of course, vary depending on the nature of the individual immune system. Some of these substances and treatments are more familiar than others, and each of them is a natural remedy and might be used in combination with other treatments, depending on your doctor's or practitioner's recommendation.

It's suggested to support these treatments with physical, emotional and spiritual exercises, as well as yoga, massage, lymphatic drainage massages, acupressure, acupuncture, light therapy and other resources which stimulate healing.

MODIFIED CITRUS PECTIN

Modified citrus pectin (MCP) is derived from the peel of citrus fruits. It's produced by an advanced modification process that alters the molecular compounds of the fruit, and thereby reduces the length of the pectin molecules, which gives MCP the properties of optimum absorption, increased bioavailability, and increased benefits for the entire body.

MCP is known to protect cellular health, support the immune system, protect against dangerous levels of toxicity, and safely remove heavy metals, while safely enhancing healthy cells.

PectaSol-C is a patented form of MCP, clinically proven to promote cellular health. The key to PectaSol-C's success is its relationship to galectin-3, a protein that causes inflammation, cardiovascular disease, and the breakdown of the cellular process. MCP binds to the galectin-3 protein, and keeps it in balance for the maintenance of health and longevity. MCP inhibits cancer from penetrating into healthy tissue. It also has a similar function as glutathione, which binds to heavy metals to eliminate them, while simultaneously supporting the immune system, without removing essential minerals like calcium, magnesium and zinc.

MCP has properties which aid in limiting disease progression in men with advanced prostate cancer. It blocks cancer cell growth, particularly with solid tumors, adhesion, angiogenesis (blood supply which feeds tumors) and metastasis. It slows PSA (prostate specific immune antibodies' marker) doubling time in the majority of patients taking a standard dose of 5 grams, 3 times per day, says Dr. Stephen Strum, an oncologist specializing in prostate cancer. Dr. Strum's vast research of MCP on several patients with prostate cancer, has shown significant results in reducing the growth and spread of tumors.

The fact that MPC releases heavy metals and does not remove healthy minerals from the body is what renders it so unique and effective. It might also prove to be another potent resource for a variety of cancer treatments. In addition, it works well in conjunction with chelation therapy.

CHELATION THERAPY

Chelation therapy is a treatment used in both conventional and alternative therapies to eliminate heavy metals and toxins from the blood. It initially began as a treatment used primarily by holistic doctors. Eventually Western practitioners caught on, acknowledging the results as effective and safe. The treatment is commonly administered intravenously utilizing a substance called ethylenediaminetetraacetic acid (EDTA), a synthetic amino acid. EDTA binds to heavy metals and minerals in the blood, eliminating them through the urine.

An oral chelation compound called Succimer, generically known as dimercaptosuccinic acid (DMSA) is FDA-approved for treatment of lead poisoning and is also used to remove mercury. Possible side effects include diarrhea, nausea, vomiting, poor appetite, or skin rash. These reactions, however, are not common. In order to minimize side effects, a client is advised to eat healthful snacks and drink plenty of water during the course of treatment.

In addition, chelation is highly effective in removing plaque from the arteries, lowering the possibility of heart attack or stroke, and reducing cholesterol levels in the blood. It offers a more affordable and less invasive procedure than bypass surgery, angioplasty, and other conventional medical treatments.

Medical doctors and alternative practitioners have stated that chelation can successfully treat vascular disease, Alzheimer's, multiple sclerosis, and other neurological disorders by reducing chemical toxicity in the body, including the brain.

The traditional intravenous treatment regimen consists of the first ten infusions delivered on a weekly basis, and the last ten delivered bi-monthly. Twenty treatments are the standard protocol, along with high doses of antioxidant vitamins and minerals that increase its efficacy.

Chelation therapy has become a more widely used treatment for detoxification of heavy metals and plaque. Some Western medical doctors, however, still question the effectiveness of chelation, in spite of the fact that numerous clinical trials have proven through X-rays and blood samples how effectively it removes toxins and plaque from the body. If your doctor tells you he doesn't believe it works or that he doesn't use the substance, get a second opinion.

It's important to check with your health care professional before undergoing chelation therapy, and to ensure that the person who administers the compound is highly qualified and certified.

PYCNOGENOL

Pycnogenol, which is pine bark from the pine tree, is known to be one of the most powerful antioxidants, with a network of over forty different antioxidant bioflavonoids. It effectively stimulates other antioxidants in the body, recycles vitamin C, and protects vitamin E from oxidation. Pycnogenol supports immunity by increasing antioxidant enzymes and glutathione, enhancing the body's ability to protect itself against free radicals. It's easily absorbed by the body (bioavailable) and improves the production of blood plasma.

Millions of dollars are spent yearly researching the functionality of this powerful super-antioxidant. French maritime pine trees, from which pycnogenol is extracted, grow exclusively along the southwest coast of France, and are processed without pesticides and toxic chemicals.

HEALTH-RELATED ISSUES THAT BENEFIT FROM PYCNOGENOL:

- Circulatory system
- Platelet growth
- Healthy blood pressure
- Helps blood move through venous system
- Reduces inflammation
- Healthy cholesterol
- Respiratory health
- Stomach comfort
- Immune response
- Brain function and memory
- Gum health
- Sunburn
- Heals wounds
- Heart health
- Diabetes control
- Menstrual symptoms
- Pregnancy hormone spikes
- Joint and muscle pain relief
- Cognitive activity
- Endurance
- Jet-lag relief

Pycnogenol can also be extracted from peanut skin, grape seed, and witch hazel bark. Over 40 years of research by the Horphag Research Company has been dedicated to establishing its quality, safety and efficacy.

GLUTAMINE

The natural healing properties of glutamine are vast and understated. After extensive research in the past fifteen years, studies show that this amino acid is a powerful element in healing the body of pathogens related to inflammation and leaky gut syndrome.

Glutamine is the most abundant amino acid in the bloodstream. Since stress depletes the body of this substance, it's important to take a glutamine supplement to support gut health and immunity.

Many people suffer from gastrointestinal disorders such as IBS, Crohn's, H. pylori, and colitis. Because of an increasing amount of toxins in the environment, we need to pay particular attention to the digestive tract. If the gut is out of balance, so is the rest of the body. Glutamine effectively strengthens and repairs the lining of the stomach and intestines.

Glutamine is excellent for relieving diarrhea because it decreases the loss of electrolytes and water from the small intestine. It's also known to support immune function, help burn patients recover from tissue damage, and increase recovery time for athletes because it supports muscle repair faster.

In Asia, glutamine is the number-one prescribed supplement for treating ulcers.

As mentioned previously, consult your professional before using glutamine.

ISATIS ROOT

Ban Lan Gen, or Isatis root, is one of the most popular traditional Chinese herbs for clinical use. It has been used in China for nearly two thousand years and contains a variety of healing properties:

- Reduces fever by killing off viruses, bacteria, and fungi
- Helps reduce the symptoms of colds and flu
- Cools the body and its fluids
- Used preventatively and curatively

During a SARS epidemic in China, Chinese herbalists used Isatis to reduce the virus, and it appeared to heal patients more effectively than other medications. Isatis is a medicinal herb from a flowering plant also known as Isatis tinctoria. Its properties are bitter and cold in nature, and relate directly to liver and stomach meridians. In Chinese medicine, bitter herbs and foods stimulate digestion and digestive juices, helping the body detoxify. A cold herb tends to cool down the body in instances of fever or toxicity.

The main functions in Chinese herbal medicine are to clear heat, cool blood, and relieve sore throat. Isatis is highly effective in clearing toxins, fever, headaches, scarlet fever, mumps, laryngitis, chickenpox, measles, hepatitis, colds, flu, meningitis, pneumonia, shingles, and herpes. It's a powerful antiviral herb, with a variety of medicinal properties.

CLINICAL WESTERN MEDICAL STUDIES SHOW IT HAS THESE ADDITIONAL FUNCTIONS:

- Detoxification
- Improvement of immune functions
- Elimination of leukemia cells

These are very significant discoveries because it indicates that Western research is stepping outside the box of traditional medicine and investigating ancient Chinese herbs and remedies, which have been used effectively for centuries to treat a variety of illnesses.

COCONUT OIL

Coconut oil has several antioxidant, immune-building, antimicrobial, antiviral, antifungal, and antibacterial properties; it contains lauric acid, capric acid, and caprylic acid, all of which are used effectively against inflammatory processes.

Coconut oil is beneficial for heart disease, diabetes, high blood pressure, HIV, cancer, autoimmune diseases, high cholesterol, weight loss, appetite reduction, immunity, candida and other fungi, viruses including colds and flu, infections, digestion, hair and skin care, stress, dental problems, and bone health.

Coconut oil contains healthful fatty acids, polyunsaturated fatty acids, monounsaturated fatty acids and polyphenols, which then become "ketones" for increased energy and cognitive function. Coconut oil also contains vitamins E and K, and helps the body absorb minerals.

Coconut oil is also therapeutic for brain disorders, including epilepsy and Alzheimer's. The fatty acids in coconut oil go directly to the liver from the digestive tract, where they are used as a source of energy. The ketones in the fatty acids are bioavailable, making coconut oil a wonderful source of nutrition for the whole body.

It's recommended to use organic virgin coconut oil for the most effective health benefits, and to eat at least one tablespoon daily in food, in a recipe, or in a healthful drink or shake.

OLIVE LEAF EXTRACT

Olive leaf extract is a potent broad-spectrum natural antimicrobial compound used to support health and eliminate infection. Olive trees and their fruit are an integral part of Mediterranean culture, both as a healthful food source and powerful medicine.

The therapeutic benefits of olive leaf extract are attributed to its bioactive compounds, called "oleuropeins." In the late 1960s, Upjohn was able to isolate ilinolic acid (an isolate of oleuropeins) and found that it was so powerful that it stopped every virus on which it was tested, including the common cold.

The antibacterial action of oleuropeins is thought to stem from its ability to dissolve pathogenic cell membranes and synthesize nitric oxide, which reduces inflammation and contributes to cellular communication.

In addition to antimicrobial and antioxidant properties, oleuropeins are shown to induce relaxation of arterial walls, reducing hypertension. A study from the University of Milan found that oleuropein inhibited oxidation of low-density lipoproteins, the bad cholesterol which is known to contribute to heart disease (It has been suggested by several more recent studies that inflammation in arterial walls causes heart disease more than high cholesterol).

Research also suggests that olive leaf extract is a potent force against immunological and bacterial disease. Olive leave extract is thought to be effective in helping the body combat a multitude of pathogens, as well as restore a deficient immune system.

Western physicians and integrative, functional doctors report that chronic fatigue and fibromyalgia patients are often helped by olive leaf extract. Studies have reported that people with autoimmune conditions attribute olive leaf extract to increased energy, minimized depression, and the elimination of many symptomatic reactions.

Olive leaf extract has antioxidant properties that help protect the body from the ubiquitous barrage of free radicals. Antioxidants neutralize free radicals (highly reactive chemical substances that might cause cellular damage within the body), viral and bacterial infections, and fungi. These properties render olive leaf extract a powerful resource for healing disease on a cellular level.

OREGANO OIL

Oregano oil has been proven in many international studies to be an effective immune booster. Compared to the herbs and plants echinacea and goldenseal, wild oil of oregano is by far the most broad-spectrum and effective natural remedy in the treatment of systemic pathogens.

ANTIBIOTIC FOR TEETH AND GUMS Oregano oil provides effective relief for toothaches by killing the bacteria that causes pain. Apply the oil directly to the infected tooth. Gum disease caused by bacteria can be arrested by using oregano oil.

ANTIFUNGAL Candida is a fungus that infects millions of people. Wild oil of oregano contains powerful antifungal agents that eliminate candida effectively and safely. The recommended doses are one to three drops under the tongue or with juice three times daily or, in more challenging cases, increased dosage by twice that amount. It's recommended to continue treatment for as long as necessary. Drink eight to ten glasses of pure spring or alkaline water daily to flush the toxins from the blood.

ANTI-INFLAMMATORY AND ANALGESIC Oregano oil has highly potent anti-inflammatory and anesthetic action. When applied externally, it deeply penetrates tissues to bring relief, speed healing, and reduce the pain of bruises, sprains, torn and sore muscles, tendonitis, cramps, carpal tunnel syndrome, and other similar injuries. Taken internally, oregano oil eliminates toxins and inflammation, reducing the pain and discomfort of arthritis.

ANTIOXIDANT Among the list of natural antioxidants, oregano oil is one of the most powerful. It protects cells from free-radical damage. Take a few drops daily in four ounces of warm water, under the tongue, to slow the effects of aging and maintain healthy cells and organs.

ANTIPARASITIC Parasites, such as head lice and scabies, may be eliminated by oregano oil's powerful antiparasitic properties. Add a few drops to a tablespoon of shampoo to wash the hair and scalp. Then add a few drops to a tablespoon of vegetable oil, and apply to the hair after shampooing. Add a whole dropper to laundry soap to disinfect clothes. Add a drop to water to protect your body from parasites such as cryptosporidium and giardia, and from bacterial infections. Ingest one to three drops up to three times daily to eliminate parasites.

ANTIVENOM Oregano oil is so potent it's capable of neutralizing venomous snake or insect bites, used both topically and orally. It's invaluable in the wilderness or when traveling to other countries. Oregano oil is also useful for preventing infection from animal bites and other puncture wounds. By applying it directly, it reduces inflammation and stops the pain associated with bites and stings. The oil penetrates the wound and neutralizes toxins and pathogens. Take a 4 or 5 drops orally 3, 4 or 5 times daily to reduce swelling or infection.

ANTIVIRAL Use daily to maintain a strong immune system and weaken viruses, including colds, flu, shingles, and herpes. At the first sign of a viral infection, immediately take three to six drops of oregano oil in four ounces of warm water. Continue taking up to three drops per hour for a maximum of ten hours. In the case of herpes or shingles, it's best to apply the oil directly to the spot where tingling is felt before an outbreak. Keep away from direct contact with genital areas.

ATHLETE'S FOOT Oregano oil is highly effective in fighting fungal infections on the feet. Rub the oil on your feet twice daily with a warm cloth until the fungus disappears.

BEDSORES Apply oregano oil topically to affected area to speed healing and reduce discomfort.

BURNS, CUTS, AND SCRAPES Apply oregano oil topically immediately, as an antibacterial, and to reduce pain and inflammation.

FOOD POISONING In a recent study, about 20 percent of meat samples obtained from grocery stores were found to contain antibiotic-resistant bacteria. Vegetarians are affected by food poisoning as well. Salmonella and E. coli are found on vegetables such as iceberg lettuce, alfalfa sprouts, and several others. Restaurant foods might be contaminated due to improper cleansing of produce. After eating, it's recommended to take three to five drops of oregano oil orally as a preventative. If symptoms of food poisoning occur, take three drops in four ounces of water hourly for up to ten hours or until symptoms disappear.

Avoid eyes, mucous membranes, and sensitive skin areas when applying wild oil of oregano.

NAIL FUNGUS Nail fungus is particularly stubborn and hard to eliminate because it's often exposed to wetness, which tends to stimulate the fungi. It's suggested that you wash and dry the nails, then soak them in wild oil of oregano twice daily for up to five minutes. Use 3 drops of oregano oil to a cup of water. Afterward, take one to three drops of the oil of oregano orally three times daily. You may continue treatment for up to six months. Nail fungus is usually a result of candida infection in the blood. Drink eight glasses of pure spring or alkaline water daily to flush the toxins from the blood.

By using oil of Oregano, you greatly reduce your chances of becoming one of the eighty-four million cases of food poisoning that occur annually in North America alone. Natural antibiotics like oil of oregano, colloidal silver and andrographis, do not induce antibiotic resistance, as do traditional antibiotic drugs. These naturally safe remedies provide highly effective defenses against biological pathogens like toxins and fungi.

WARTS Use a cotton ball to apply oil of oregano directly to the wart. Leave the soaked cotton on the wart for as long as possible by covering it with an adhesive bandage. Repeat this two or three times a day. Since warts are viral, take three drops under the tongue three times a day for a few months. Plantar warts can be successfully removed in a few days by applying the oil directly to the skin several times daily.

It's important to note that when you kill these pathogens, they release toxins into the bloodstream.

The toxins might cause fatigue, flu or cold symptoms, and in some cases, skin rashes. If you develop a rash, it's a sign that your body is trying to detoxify. Since your skin is the largest organ in the body, rashes, hives, or skin irritations are a natural progression of detoxification.

Any of these reactions are known as a healing crisis, or a Herxheimer reaction. Avoid discomfort by drinking eight to twelve glasses of pure spring water daily. Water flushes toxins from your blood, and might alleviate "die-off" reactions.

Because we are all completely individual in body chemistry, there's no one specific dosage for everyone. A small amount of trial-and-error might be necessary to determine the optimum dosage level for your particular condition. Listen to your body; it's your best gauge. Some people require less than recommended dosages, while others need up to two or three times that.

In these cases, spread extra doses over the period of a day rather than taking them all at once. For example, take three drops ten times daily rather than ten drops three times daily.

Oregano oil has been laboratory tested and proven to be as strong as pharmaceutical antibiotics with none of the associated side-effects. It's highly effective both topically and internally for a variety of infections.

ANDROGRAPHIS

Andrographis paniculata is an herb used extensively in India and China, but rarely, if ever, recognized in modern Western medicinal practice. It's a fairly uncommon and unknown herbal remedy, but the curative effects are potent and worthy of note.

This medicinal plant, also known as Chuan Xin Lian, or Chirata, is grown widely in the tropics and subtropics, and used in Asia for a variety of conditions, including fever, flu, and gastrointestinal pathogens such as dysentery, hepatitis, stomach ulcers, colitis, respiratory diseases, allergies, venomous snake and scorpion bites, malaria, ear and skin infections, and vaginitis.

Traditional Chinese medicine describes the properties of andrographis to be good for clearing heat and, therefore, known for eliminating toxins and fever. There is an increased interest in andrographis because it's easily cultivated, and offers relief for the treatments of inflammation, bacteria, virus and cancer.

A drop on the gums is believed to stimulate saliva and digestive enzymes. There's scientific evidence from clinical trials that indicates its powerful effect on the gastrointestinal system. Studies also show andrographis protects the liver from toxins, and the stomach from ulceration by inflammation and disease.

A BRIEF SUMMARY OF CURRENT RESEARCH AND TRIALS INCLUDES THESE FINDINGS:

- Andrographis kills and repels mosquitoes that transmit malaria.
- Studies show the herb has antiviral activity against dengue fever, which means that with more research, the world might gain additional alternatives to treat this often deadly disease.
- Researchers have identified anti-herpes virus qualities.

Laboratory research also shows it might have useful applications in the treatment of asthma and respiratory inflammation. One fairly recent study demonstrated that a component of this herb might combat the progressive debilitation of rheumatoid arthritis (RA). Considering the number of people who suffer from RA, this is a significant and important discovery.

When birds were fed a mixture of several herbs, including andrographis, the toxic effect of heavy metals from the environment were minimized and tended to accumulate less in their bodies.

COLLOIDAL SILVER

Colloidal silver is one of the oldest remedies in the world, but is little known and undervalued in the medical model. Its uses are so varied, medically documented, and highly effective for supporting the body's immune system, that it's surprising there is such little research.

At the very least, its ability to purify water anywhere in the world makes it crucially important, particularly in poorer countries where contamination is so prevalent.

Experts in the study of colloidal silver consider it to be one of the most effective defenses against emerging strains of pathogens. It attacks bacterial, viral, and fungal infections. Whether it's used topically, for immune support during acute flu or colds, or for preventive purposes, colloidal silver is a versatile and broad-spectrum holistic compound.

Consumers should be selective and informed. Some colloidal silver products are not high in quality—the particulate matter clog together and, therefore, have little surface area or valuable activity. In addition, some companies use preservatives or additives that coat the silver particles and reduce its efficacy.

THE MANY USES OF COLLOIDAL SILVER:

- **CANDIDA ALBICANS** Swallow one tablespoon of silver with one tablespoon of aloe vera juice on an empty stomach three times per day. Follow treatment for two weeks.

- **COLDS OR FLU** Hold one to two teaspoons under tongue for thirty seconds, and swallow. Repeat every few hours, preferably on an empty stomach.

- **EAR INFECTIONS** Four drops in the ear, leave for two minutes, then drain out. Repeat three to four times per day.

- **EYE INFECTIONS** Two drops in the eye, three to four times per day to treat pink eye or conjunctivitis.

- **FOOD POISONING OR DYSENTERY** Swallow one table-spoon directly, every hour, without holding under tongue. Take on an empty stomach.

- **FOOT ODOR** Spray feet and toes in the morning and at night.

- **MINOR SKIN INJURIES** Five sprays directly on problem area such as a cut, scrape, burn, or infection. Repeat five times per day.

- **MOUTH AND GUM INFECTIONS** Hold one teaspoon on area inside mouth for a few minutes, then swallow. Repeat three to four times a day.

- **NAIL FUNGUS** Spray or drop on area several times a day.

- **NASAL INFECTIONS** One dropper into each nostril while sitting with head tilted forward to access sinus cavities. Leave in for two minutes, then swallow. Repeat three times per day.

- **RESPIRATORY INFECTIONS** Place one teaspoon in a nebulizer and inhale for ten minutes. Repeat three times per day.

- **SORE THROAT OR STREP** Gargle one tablespoon for two minutes, and swallow. Repeat five times per day.

- **TRAVELER'S DIARRHEA** Swallow one teaspoon three to seven times per day for a few days.

- **URINARY TRACT INFECTION** See directions for food poisoning.

- **VAGINAL INFECTIONS** Mix one part silver and two parts distilled water. Hold inside vagina for a few minutes. Repeat two times per day.

- **WATER PURIFICATION** Drop into water, one to two tablespoons per gallon of water.

These are only some of the natural treatments utilized for a host of autoimmune diseases. They are effective when used individually, or may be used in combination with one another, depending on your doctor's recommendation.

All of these remedies are effective in conjunction with other physical, emotional and spiritual practices, as they all work synergistically for optimum healing. It's significant to emphasize that, as always, healing is an inside job, and attitude, mind-set, faith and belief systems, all work together to help the body heal.

CHAPTER 8

CHINESE HERBS AND THEIR FUNCTIONS

It's estimated that about five thousand plant species are used for medicinal purposes, and many are also consumed for their nutritional value. The acceptance of herbal medicine in the West owes a great debt to Asian cultures, which have used herbs as remedies for thousands of years. Some of these plants are well-known in this country, like ginseng, honeysuckle, licorice, jasmine, reishi mushroom, and many others.

Think of herbs as food, each herb having its own function in supporting the immune system. They are as varied and they are numerous, and it's important to understand the properties, functions, principles, patterns and channels which each herb addresses. This knowledge helps you in your healing process, and supports a positive outcome.

The **principles** of traditional Chinese medicine are based on energy meridians, acupuncture, and herbal supplements. In America, this was originally practiced as "folk medicine," and today, some of the plants are used in traditional Western medicine. The roots of herbal plants are the most important parts, followed by the seeds and fruits.

The four **properties** of herbs are cold, hot, warm, and cool, and the standard procedure is to treat heat conditions, like fever and infections, with cold-natured herbs, and the opposite for cold conditions. The theory in herbal medicine is to cool down a hot body and warm up a cold body or condition. Each condition has a unique property: for instance, fever is considered to be "hot," since it raises the temperature of the body. Therefore, a "cold" herb, or an herb used to cool down the body, is indicated. The herb itself has no temperature, but rather, has properties which can either cool or heat a specific condition. A cold condition is in someone who is naturally cold, and therefore, needs warmer herbs, or hot teas, to balance the body.

There are five **flavors** of herbs: sour, bitter, sweet, hot, and salty. Hot expels cold, sour is like an astringent or poultice, sweet is for pain, bitter helps dry tissue (such as dampness in the stomach from diarrhea), and salty softens lumps such as tumors. Some herbal remedies have more than one flavor and action, depending on the pathology. These flavors work in conjunction with the properties of heat and cold, and damp and dry. The choices of herbs are dependent on the condition at hand.

There are also **patterns** in herbal functions, such as lifting, lowering, floating, and sinking, that are measured by feeling the activity of the pulse. This is determined by the nature of the pulse, which then determines the nature of the condition. The theory in Chinese medicine is to utilize an herb that moves in the opposite direction of the disorder—this is how disease is treated. For example, if the pulse is slow and "thready" (feels like a rope to the touch), the herb used would be to quicken the energy in the body and smooth the thready condition. A Chinese practitioner will be qualified to discern which herb is necessary to treat a condition, depending on the movement of the pulse.

There are also **channels** that govern a particular meridian, organ, or group of organs on which a particular herb has an effect. They are specific and part of the education of Chinese herbology. The area of the body, organ or energetic system is evaluated when determining herbs or herbal combinations.

THE FOLLOWING IS A PARTIAL LIST OF SOME COMMONLY USED CHINESE HERBS, THEIR ACTIONS, AND HOW THEY AFFECT VARIOUS CONDITIONS:

ACANTHOPANAX ROOT BARK—acts as effective heart tonic; relieves pain and rheumatism; treats diarrhea; reduces inflammation

ANDROGRAPHIS—alleviates bacterial infections; detoxifies, supports immunity and respiratory tract; helps normalize body temperature; reduces stress and supports liver function

ANGELICA ROOT—treats heartburn; gas, loss of appetite, anti-spasmodic, menopause symptoms; PMS, allergies, sinuses, nerves and insomnia

APRICOT SEED (B17)—relieves dry cough; asthma, constipation and has been used to treat cancer

ASIAN DANDELION—antibacterial properties treat mastitis; hepatitis, appendicitis, gall bladder, jaundice, constipation, edema and inflammation; cirrhosis of the liver; urinary infection; tonsillitis, laryngitis, and common cold

ASTRAGALUS ROOT—improves energy; stimulates immune system during colds, flu, blood disorders, cancer, HIV virus, and bacteria; improves adrenals and digestion; treats bladder infections, blood sugar and metabolism; boosts natural interferon; protects kidneys; increases resistance to stress; helps balance the body.

BLACK COHOSH—helps with arthritis; fibromyalgia, depression, menopausal symptoms; menstrual cramps and PMS; lowers blood pressure and cholesterol; treats rattlesnake bites as an anti-venom

BOSWELLIA—helps with bursitis; inflammation, arthritis, injuries, ulcerative colitis; Crohn's, IBS, and asthma

BUPLEURUM—treats pneumonia; flu, bronchitis, indigestion, fever, cough, muscle pain; cramps, depression, and headache; clears liver toxins; strengthens immunity

CALENDULA—applied topically helps heal cuts, scrapes, rashes, and burns

CAYENNE—improves circulation; serves as an antiseptic; induces sweat to eliminate toxins; treats fevers, asthma, varicose veins, colic, gas, and laryngitis; soothes sore throats; relieves pain

CHINESE EPHEDRA—decreases hunger and pain; opens lungs; treats asthma, allergies, hay fever, weakness in kidneys; excessive perspiration, and night sweats

CHINESE PULSATILLA—relieves dysentery; nosebleeds and swelling; helps alleviate depression; clears gut toxins, wounds, and viral infections

CHINESE YAM—strengthens spleen, stomach, digestion, and immune system; nourishes blood; relieves diarrhea and vaginal discharge; helps balance blood sugar

CINNAMON BARK—relieves stomach upset, diarrhea, and gas; supports the lymphatic system; treats infections from bacteria or parasites; treats colds and flu; balances blood sugar (excellent for diabetics)

CLOVES—relieves nausea and indigestion; kills parasites; reduces allergies; kills bacteria and fungus; soothes toothache

COMFREY—treats ulcers; colitis, IBS and Crohn's; bronchitis; inflammation, muscle aches; psoriasis, eczema, and wounds

CORIANDER—treats stomach disorders; inflammation, and burns; detoxifies; boosts memory; gives spleen support; has a laxative effect

CYPRESS KERNEL—nourishes heart, kidneys, and large intestine; treats heart palpitations; insomnia, constipation, and night sweats

DAMIANA—clears urinary tract infection; acts as a diuretic; helps treat depression, digestion; hormone balance; anxiety, and PMS

DANGGUI—protects liver; tones blood; regulates menstruation and PMS; helps balance hormones

DEVIL'S CLAW—reduces hardening of the arteries; treats back and muscle pain; tendonitis, chest pain, gastrointestinal upset; menstrual cramps, and migraines

ECHINACEA AND ELDERBERRY—help colds; flu, cough, sore throat; support immune system; antiviral and antibacterial; and helps sinusitis

ELEUTHERO (Siberian Ginseng)—relieves stress and anxiety; detoxifies; treats menopause and hormone balance

EUCALYPTUS—used externally, clears lungs; bronchial passages and nasal passages; treats respiratory disease; colds, flu, and sinus infections

FENNEL—antimicrobial; aids in digestion; treats gas, colic, spasms; respiratory infections; urinary tract infections; PMS; reduces stress

FENUGREEK—helps with digestive tract inflammation; colic; blood sugar imbalances; increases breast milk supply; reduces high cholesterol and fever, skin inflammation and constipation

FLAX—helps IBS and spastic colon; bronchitis; PMS; eczema; arthritis, plant estrogen and antioxidant properties; inflammation; source of protein and fiber

FEVERFEW—soothes migraines and other headaches; reduces fever, treats digestive problems; arthritis

FRANKINCENSE—used as antiseptic; acts as a sedative; improves circulation; treats pain, PMS, and urinary tract infections; dries phlegm

GANODERMA—effective for asthma; anti-cancer effects; supports heart and liver; stimulates white blood cells and immunity; has calming effects; can relieve pain

GARLIC—treats viral, fungal and bacterial infections; lowers blood pressure, cholesterol, and fever; relieves cough; detoxifies; reduces perspiration

GENTIAN ROOT—helps digestion; treats gas; increases appetite; supports liver, stimulates saliva

GINGER—detoxifies from food poisoning; reduces gas; helps colds, nausea, and bronchitis; is anti-inflammatory; stimulates digestion

GINKGO BILOBA—helps memory; treats attention deficit disorder (ADD) and attention deficit hyperactivity disorder (ADHD); improves circulation; treats depression, high blood pressure; PMS; radiation toxicity; tinnitus; helps stroke recovery; macular degeneration; vertigo, and migraines

GINSENG—tones the lungs; increases energy; nourishes stomach; promotes fluids, clears heat; lowers blood sugar and cholesterol; reduces stress; treats male sexual function

GOLDENSEAL—aids in digestion; increases appetite; treats diarrhea; sinuses; viral and bacterial infections; PMS, and bleeding

GOTU KOLA—has antianxiety and anti-stress properties; improves circulation, memory, and concentration; helps veins; promotes hair and nail growth; stimulates collagen

GRAPEFRUIT SEED—detoxifies blood; has antiviral, antifungal, and antibacterial actions; treats upset stomach; calms nervous system

GYMNEMA SYLVESTRE—helps insulin balance and diabetes; weight loss; malaria; cough; diuretic

HAWTHORN—effective heart tonic; improves circulation; lowers blood pressure; aids digestion; reduces possibility of congestive heart failure

HEMP SEED—high in antioxidants and minerals; anti-inflammatory actions; lowers blood pressure; stimulates skin, hair growth; regulates metabolism; helps brain function; moisturizing

HOLY BASIL—lowers cholesterol; has anticancer, antibacterial, antianxiety, anti-depression, and antioxidant properties; controls blood sugar; protects heart

HORSE CHESTNUT—stimulates circulation; reduces swelling in legs, fatigue; diuretic; arterial sclerosis; veins; inflammation, and heart

HYSSOP—treats colds; respiratory and bronchial infections; cough; bruises, and abrasions

ISATIS ROOT—has excellent antiviral and antibacterial properties; treats colds, flu, and mumps; cools the body, reduces fever

IVY—external use treats skin conditions; warts, fungus, inflammation, and toothache

JAPANESE HONEYSUCKLE—protects liver; relieves flu symptoms; treats mumps; reduces fat in blood; acts as an antibacterial agent

JIU WEI TAI (Stomach Peace)—treats stomach problems; pain; nausea; IBS, and reflux; acts as an anti-inflammatory

JUNIPER—helps with cystitis; kidney conditions; arthritis; gout; indigestion; gas, and bloating

KAVA—treats insomnia; depression; mood swings; hyperactivity; anxiety, and muscle spasms

KUDZU VINE—expands coronary arteries; reduces heat; treats blood pressure; relieves alcoholic cravings; lowers blood sugar

LEMONGRASS—soothes muscle spasms; anxiety; exhaustion, and digestion; insomnia; respiratory disorders; fever; edema; cellular health; maintains healthy cholesterol; balances blood sugar

LICORICE—tones spleen and stomach; helps dry cough; stomach pain; swelling, and food poisoning; harmonizes various herbs; supports immunity

LINDEN FLOWERS—used for colds; muscle spasms; flu; high blood pressure; headache; digestion, and calming

LOMATIUM—offers immune support; has antiviral and antibacterial effects; treats colds, flu, bronchitis and urinary tract infections; diuretic

LYCIUM FRUIT (Goji)—antioxidant; boosts immunity; tones kidneys; nourishes liver; helps dizziness; depression; inflammation; anemia; cough; eye irritations; vertigo; blurred vision, and high blood pressure; acts as sedative; arrests vomiting; aids longevity

MACA—increases stamina and energy; promotes hormone balance and mental clarity; treats anxiety and depression; reduces blood pressure; blocks production of cancer cells; might increase libido

MAGNOLIA—relieves sinusitis and headache; opens nasal passages; indigestion, gas, nausea and menstrual cramps; treats coughs and asthma

MAITAKE MUSHROOM—has anticancer properties; helps with chronic fatigue syndrome; autoimmune disorders; colds, and flu; stimulates immunity; may control blood sugar, high cholesterol and blood pressure; used to treat HIV/AIDS

MARSHMALLOW—treats nausea; inflammation; respiratory problems; cough, bronchitis; digestion, and skin inflammation

MILK THISTLE—helps clean liver; treats cirrhosis, hepatitis, gallstones, alcohol and drug addiction; PMS; indigestion; skin conditions such as eczema and acne

MISTLETOE—nourishes blood; helps weak legs; opens arteries; lowers blood pressure; relieves pain; treats flu; epilepsy; arthritis; hypertension; inflammation

MORINDA ROOT—treats impotence and reproductive organs; low back pain; liver repair; pain in stomach; weakness in knees and low back, and rheumatism due to kidney deficiency; possible cancer and heart disease prevention; lowers blood sugar; supports immunity

MOTHERWORT—strengthens uterus; increases milk supply; relieves angina; lowers thyroid; regulates PMS and aids reproduction; treats heart palpitations; inflammation

MSM—reduces allergies; aids bones; relieves muscle and joint pain; helps digest protein and fats; treats inflammation, depression and cancer; improves skin and hair; improves energy; detoxifying; stimulates immunity

MYRRH—helps respiratory and stomach problems; anti-inflammatory, antimicrobial, antifungal; expectorant; stimulates immunity; supports circulation; rejuvenates energy

NEROLI—treats indigestion, heartburn, and gas; boosts appetite; reduces bloating; antiseptic; antidepressant; antibacterial; disinfectant; supports digestion; sedative;

OAT STRAW—treats shingles, herpes; menopause, depression, and anxiety; boosts immunity; supports longevity; improves cognition; stimulates cell growth and bones; strengthens blood vessels

PASSION FLOWER—treats insomnia; anxiety, digestion, and drug withdrawal; high blood pressure

PINELLIA—treats nausea, morning sickness; coughs, flu, pain, and swelling

PUMPKIN SEED—treats parasites; boosts immunity; reduces enlarged prostate; antioxidants; supports heart (magnesium); supports healthy menopause; improves insulin regulation; sleep aid; anti-inflammatory

RADIX REHMANNIAE—acts on heart; liver, and kidney meridians; clears body heat; cools blood; lubricates intestines; produces fluids

REISHI—treats respiratory, heart, and liver issues; lowers blood pressure and cholesterol; has anticancer properties; boosts immunity; treats bacterial infections, stress, and anxiety

RESVERATROL—treats immune deficiency; has antiviral, anti-inflammatory and antibacterial properties; protects arteries for blood flow; reduces stress; protects against heart disease and possibly cancer

RHUBARB—relieves constipation; helps gall bladder; clears bacteria; antioxidant; supports bone growth and neuronal damage to brain; supports eyes and vision

SAGE—treats gas; sweating; depression, and anxiety; improves liver function; antioxidant; calming; supports memory; antifungal, antibacterial; soothes digestion

SAW PLAMETTO—treats respiratory inflammation; sore throat and bronchitis; asthma; increases libido; reduces prostate swelling; strengthens kidneys, bladder, and immunity;

SLIPPERY ELM—soothes membranes of respiratory tract, and digestive and urinary tracts; treats bronchitis; colitis, ulcers, heartburn, gastritis; sore throats, and bladder infections

ST. JOHN'S WORT—taken internally treats anxiety, depression, seasonal affective disorder (SAD), and viruses; topically treats burns, scrapes, nerve pain, and bruises

STINGING NETTLE—builds blood; treats PMS, kidney stones, and lung problems; promotes proteins in the body; full of valuable nutrients; detoxifies; relieves allergies and arthritis

THYME—treats coughs, respiratory infections; mucus, gas, inflammation, and tonsillitis; lowers blood pressure and cholesterol; boosts immunity; disinfectant

TURMERIC—has anti-inflammatory and anticancer properties; relieves arthritis pain; increases circulation; supports stomach and gall bladder; treats PMS, liver disorders, asthma, depression, and indigestion

URVA URSI—treats cystitis, urinary infections; candida, and inflammation

VALERIAN—helps relieve insomnia; restlessness; spasms, and pain

WHITE WILLOW BARK—ingredient in aspirin; used to relieve pain, inflammation, muscle aches, headaches, and other inflammatory ailments; relieves acne and menstrual cramps

WILD DATE (Jujube)—tones liver and kidneys; soothes skin conditions; has sedative and laxative properties; reduces blood sugar levels; antioxidant

WORMWOOD—helps rid body of parasites, reduces indigestion; supports liver and gall bladder function

YARROW—induces sweat to break fevers; treats toothache, digestive problems, IBS, and circulation

YELLOW DOCK—soothes sore throat; helps iron deficiency (anemia); serves as a liver tonic; detoxifying; anti-inflammation; anti-bacterial; laxative

YIN CHIAO—reduces symptoms and pathogens of colds and flu, such as fever, aches, runny nose, and fatigue

There are many, many more Chinese herbs and herbal formulas that work in conjunction with one another. A qualified Chinese herbalist, naturopath, or holistic practitioner can recommend herbs and combinations according to the specific disorder.

It's recommended to check in with a professional before attempting to take herbs on your own.

Some herbs are contraindicated with certain medications. Herbal remedies have been used for healing purposes for centuries, are popular in various countries all over the world, have cured many people of a variety of illnesses, and have powerful nutritional properties.

CONTROVERSIAL CANNABIDIOL:
A compound called cannabidiol, from the marijuana plant, is an herb which does not create a "high" and is particularly helpful in treating certain medical conditions. Because it is non-psychoactive, it has few side effects and is used to treat even small children

to control epilepsy. It has other natural medicinal properties that have become increasingly valuable to the health care community:

- Antianxiety
- Antidepressant
- Anticancer
- Anti-inflammatory
- Anti-nausea
- Antioxidant
- Anti-psychotic

Unfortunately, cannabidiol, which is surrounded by controversy, is currently illegal in many states. In the most serious cases of epilepsy, especially in children, some parents are not able at this time to treat their children with this potent herb. More legislation is necessary to legalize cannabidiol in more states, and worldwide.

As an example, a couple who lived in New Jersey and have a little girl with severe epilepsy, were forced to move to Oregon (where cannabidiol is legal) to treat their child. They stated that the use of this herb reduced the child's seizures by more than half, undeniably saving her life.

Case studies and reports indicate numerous beneficial supplemental, nutrient-rich, and phytochemical compounds derived from the marijuana plant. Although there is much controversy about its use, derivatives of the marijuana plant might prove to have a potent effect on specific health challenges, including cancer.

HOME REMEDIES FOR IMMUNE-RELATED CONDITIONS

The following is a list of natural health remedies for home-use. This list is simple, straight-forward and practical. The supplements and herbs all relate to the immune system, and are substances suggested to minimize the effects of symptoms without, in some cases, seeing a specialist or holistic practitioner.

These suggestions can save money, time, aggravation and a lot of driving; you can decide for yourselves what works best for you.

The most effective treatment is to try 1 or 2 protocols at a time, and not to do all of them at once. If you aren't sure or have any questions about directions, contraindications with medications, allergies or any other issues, it's best to consult with a practitioner who is knowledgeable in natural medicine. In most cases, you can follow the directions on the label for amounts and millegrams to be taken.

Obviously, if your condition is serious, life-threatening, or dire, you'd be advised to see a medical specialist.

ACNE Avoid dairy and fried, greasy foods; reduce oily makeup; reduce amounts of sugar and sodas; keep your hands off your face, and do not pick or squeeze; avoid sun; evaluate your birth control (might cause acne); use one acne medicine at a time, or use natural drying agents; get allergy tested.

ALLERGIES Get allergy tested; keep air vents in house and car clean; get an air purifier; seal your bed and pillows with allergy covers; keep humidity out of your house (creates mold and fungus); bathe your pets; get herbal allergy remedies at your local health food store (Chinese herb, Bi Yan Pian, is very effective).

ANGINA (Chest Pain) Eat light meals several times a day; avoid smoking and excessive alcohol; use daily supplements such as CoQ10, magnesium, bromelain, arginine and carnitine (unless contra-indicated); hawthorn, propolis, red sage, lobelia, cayenne (circulation), and licorice root.

ATHLETE'S FOOT Keep feet dry and clean; soak them in warm saltwater; apply coconut oil or tea tree oil; swab with olive oil and colloidal silver (antifungal); eat alfalfa, ginger, and garlic; avoid sugar, sodas, dairy, and acidic foods (see candida diet in Chapter 2).

ARTHRITIS Detoxify (arthritis is primarily caused by toxins in the joints); stretch your muscles; take natural anti-inflammation remedies, like boswellia, turmeric, and white willow bark; rub joints in warm eucalyptus oil; use ice to reduce inflammation; boost vitamin C and fish oil intake; get massages; reduce foods that cause inflammation, like sugar, gluten and alcohol.

ASTHMA Avoid cigarette smoke and known allergies; elevate your head when sleeping; keep neck covered during cold weather; do breathing exercises to increase lung capacity; beware of food additives; take caffeine in moderation (dilates capillaries as it opens lungs); take antioxidant supplements; get natural herbal and homeopathic inhalers (local health food stores).

BACKACHE Elevate legs; do low back stretches; swim; use ice or moist heat; sleep with knee pillow; take white willow bark for pain;

hang upside down to stretch vertebrae; try yoga or Pilates; get a good mattress, ergonomic chairs, and car seats; take zinc, copper, boron, MSM, glucosamine-chondroitin, devil's claw, boswellia, and turmeric to reduce inflammation (take two or three only during painful episodes).

BLADDER INFECTIONS Drink lots of fluids and unsweetened cranberry juice; detoxify; empty bladder before and after sex; avoid acidic foods and liquids; eat alkaline foods and beverages.

BLOOD PRESSURE Avoid weight gain; reduce salt and alcohol intake; take potassium (if indicated by doctor); eat a more vegetarian diet; do low impact exercise; avoid stress; take fish oil, B complex, hawthorn berry herb, CoQ10, and magnesium; eat organic foods, like beets, greens, and squash; avoid processed foods.

BREAST DISCOMFORT Low-fat, high-fiber diet; take vitamins C, B complex, magnesium, and E; take maca powder and herb dong quai to balance hormones; massage your breasts; use light scrub to stimulate lymph glands; check breasts for lumps; avoid caffeine, dairy, sugar, and birth control pills.

BRONCHITIS Avoid smoking; drink lots of fluids; steam your lungs with eucalyptus oil or plain water; avoid dairy (causes mucus); use natural herbs and remedies such as slippery elm, licorice root, mullein, ginger, and wild cherry bark; drink honey-lemon tea; take colloidal silver and andrographis, or isatis root to reduce infection.

BRUXISM (Teeth Grinding) Release stress; avoid caffeine, sugar, chocolate-- especially before sleep (chocolate has caffeine) and dairy; take B-complex, magnesium, potassium, SAM-e, tyrosine, zinc, chromium; hops, passion flower, lemon balm, valerian, 5-HTP, and melatonin.

BURSITIS Avoid acidic foods; detoxify and alkaline the body with raw celery, apple cider vinegar, carrot juice; burdock tea, turmeric, boswellia, ginger, flaxseed oil, vitamin C, and bromelain; use a warm castor oil compress on inflammation for releasing toxins.

CARPAL TUNNEL SYNDROME Rotate hand in circles for light stretching; take B6 and anti-inflammation herbs like boswellia, turmeric, and white willow bark; use ice pack and wrist brace; get massages; avoid activities that cause inflammation.

CELLULITE Eat green foods; avoid sugar, caffeine, sodas, fatty fried food, and dairy; eat fiber; get lymphatic massages; drink lots of water; eliminate salt; get plenty of exercise; take ginger, artichoke extract, dandelion root, garlic, ginseng, pumpkin seed barley, oats, fish oil, red yeast rice; niacin, fiber, and fenugreek (blood cleanse); detoxify.

COLDS Take vitamin C, zinc, ginger, and garlic; drink fluids; eat chicken soup; take goldenseal, echinacea, isatis root tea (or tincture), colloidal silver, oregano oil, olive leaf extract; steam with eucalyptus oil and water; avoid dairy and sugar; drink tea with honey, cinnamon, ginger, garlic, and cayenne.

COLD SORES Keep sore clean and dry; use zinc topically and orally; take lysine and vitamin C; use vanilla extract and peppermint oil topically; drink licorice tea; avoid chocolate, caffeine, peas, grains, peanuts, cashews (rich in arginine which feeds virus), and alcohol.

CONJUNCITVITIS Soak eyes externally with warm baking soda and water; take probiotics; use cool tea bags on eyes for inflammation; make a soak of one teaspoon each: comfrey, raspberry, and goldenseal with one cup of boiling water, steep for an hour, cool until warm, and use with dropper into eye; take echinacea, colloidal silver, oregano oil, elderberry tincture (supports immunity), and vitamins C, A, and B-complex.

CONSTIPATION Drink lots of water; take magnesium and fiber; exercise; avoid dairy; take herbs and other natural remedies like senna, cascara, rhubarb, licorice extract, and aloe juice; get tested for candida and parasites.

DEPRESSION Exercise; take St. John's wort, L-tyrosine, B-complex, Q96, Protandim, folic acid, 5-HTP, MSM, ginkgo, GABA, omega-3, SAM-e, and magnesium; avoid sugar and dairy; get acupuncture and massage; meditate; try light therapy (see specialist if severe).

DERMATITIS AND ECZEMA Avoid dairy, sugar, acidic foods, coffee, and alcohol; do candida cleanse diet to clear rashes and eczema; take evening primrose oil, zinc, B-complex, vitamin E, acidophilus; do a kelp and bentonite soak; apply coconut oil or aloe gel on skin; make a tea of calendula, marigold flowers, and lavender, and apply to skin; detoxify body (Skin conditions usually originate in the gut).

DIABETES Consume cinnamon, ginger, fenugreek, bilberry, cloves, curry, guava, aloe, apple cider vinegar, bilberry, oats, garlic, onions, basil, fig leaves; CoQ10, zinc, magnesium, chromium, niacin, B-complex, garlic, ginseng, and fiber (see a specialist); avoid sugars and fats; lower cholesterol.

DIVERTICULOSIS Chew foods well; drink fluids; eat fiber; avoid dairy and processed foods, nuts, and seeds; avoid caffeine and alcohol; take broad-spectrum probiotics, vitamins C and B, garlic, alfalfa, aloe vera juice, glutamine, glutathione, apple cider vinegar; colloidal silver, oregano oil, and olive leaf extract; detoxify.

EAR INFECTION Try NutriBiotic Ear Drops and nasal spray (Whole Foods Market carries it); avoid dairy and sugar; put a few drops of warm olive oil in ear with cotton ball; take vitamin C, colloidal silver, and garlic; put a few drops of warm mullein oil into ear; use immune-boosting herbs such as astragalus, echinacea, ginseng, cat's claw, and antioxidant supplements.

EAR WAX Put full dropper of warm olive oil, garlic oil, or hydrogen peroxide (small amount) into ear, lay on opposite side for five minutes while wax softens, then let oil drain out of ear—wax should exit with it (if not, repeat procedure).

EMPHYSEMA, PULMONARY FIBROSIS, COPD Avoid secondhand smoke and allergens; do breathing exercises or yoga; eat little and often; breathe from your diaphragm; take vitamins C and E; avoid sprays and toxic products; take Neprinol (breaks up fibrous tissue in lungs) and Tibetan Herbal Balance Lung Support (go to Biogetica.com, and check out T26 Lung Liquescence and C84 Anti-Scar Formula).

Contrary to Western medical model, fibrosis, or fibrous tissue, might be eliminated in some cases.

ENDOMETRIOSIS Reduce eating foods with animal fats; eat broccoli, cauliflower, Brussels sprouts, kale, flaxseed, celery, and parsley; take ashwagandha, dong quai, maca powder; goldenseal, milk thistle (liver), chasteberry; omega-3, vitamins C, B vitamins, folic acid, zinc, and magnesium.

EXTREME FATIGUE Get blood work; drink green juice and lots of water; eat superfoods like kale, spinach, moringa powder, chlorella, spirulina, maca; cabbage, broccoli, sprouts, carrots, apples, cucumber, ginger, and garlic; take vitamins C, E, B's, D3, and omegas; reduce red meats; avoid wheat, dairy, sugar, and caffeine (drink green tea for energy); eat brown rice, quinoa, legumes, millet, and kamut.

FLATULENCE (Gas) Avoid gassy foods such as dairy, fried foods, carbonated beverages, cabbage, broccoli, onions, radishes, and fruits such as apricots and bananas; take charcoal tablets; drink peppermint and chamomile teas; use turmeric, fennel, anise, caraway, and coriander.

FLU Avoid sugar, caffeine, white flour, and dairy (all cause inflammation and mucous); take vitamins C, D3, B's, and zinc; take oregano oil (reduces infection), olive leaf extract, organic germanium, echinacea, isatis root (or tincture), apple cider vinegar, and colloidal silver; steam nose with eucalyptus oil; drink lots of water and warm teas.

FOOD POISONING Avoid uncooked meats and eggs; eat shellfish only if it's fresh; avoid sushi; drink strong ginger, peppermint, and chamomile teas; use rosemary, fenugreek, and holy basil; drink warm water with lemon; take activated charcoal tablets; put three tablespoons of apple cider vinegar in warm water, and *sip* three times a day.

FORGETFULNESS Take omega-3, betacarotene, folic acid, B12, rhodiola, bacopa (for anxiety and blood pressure), GABA, gotu kola, ginkgo biloba, ashwagandha, turmeric, ginseng, sage, green tea, periwinkle, rosemary, peppermint, basil, schisandra, and blueberries.

GENITAL HERPES Take vitamin C, B vitamins, L-Lysine, zinc, echinacea and goldenseal (fight virus), H-Plex Defense (name of product); burdock root (for blisters), prunella, Rozites (mushrooms that fight virus); colloidal silver, oregano oil, olive leaf extract, isatis herb; propolis, calendula, and black seed ointment (topically).

HANGOVER Drink lots of water; absorb alcohol with saltines or bread; take vitamin C, amino acids, B-complex; evening primrose, peppermint, white willow bark, chicory, milk thistle; magnesium, fennel, carrots (clean liver), fenugreek, ginger, or thyme.

HEADACHES Take white willow bark, ashwagandha, feverfew, ginger, ginkgo biloba; caffeine, guarana (opens capillaries), chamomile, valerian; magnesium, B6, B2, omegas, and CoQ10; drink water; detoxify.

HEARTBURN Avoid coffee, sodas, and acidic foods; take charcoal, papaya digestive enzymes, apple cider vinegar (alkalizes acids); ginger root, bitters (herbs), catnip, probiotics, licorice, and fennel.

HEMORRHOIDS Make teas or ointments for topical use that include nettle, elderberry, comfrey, myrrh, yarrow, calendula cream, aloe gel, mullein and witch hazel; detoxify; take natural laxatives such as senna, flax, licorice, rhubarb, or dried fruit.

INSOMNIA Avoid sugar, chocolate, and caffeine after 2:00 p.m.; take melatonin, valerian root, scullcap, L-theanine, tryptophan, 5-HTP, California poppy, passion flower, hops, chamomile, catnip (herbal), or kava kava; take adrenal supplement to calm cortisol levels; listen to "white noise;" take lavender baths; get massages; try acupuncture.

IRRITABLE BOWEL SYNDROME Avoid dairy, coffee, acidic foods, roughage, and alcohol; take probiotics, glutamine, glutathione, and digestive enzymes; drink lots of water; take natural fiber, peppermint tea or oil, chamomile tea, slippery elm, cinnamon, cardamom, ginger, and fennel; detoxify.

KIDNEY STONES Avoid foods high in uric acid like caffeine, chocolate, oranges, and sugar; take zinc, potassium, magnesium citrate; chanca piedra (herb that breaks up stones), watermelon, cranberry juice, pomegranate juice, celery, apple cider vinegar, olive oil, lemon juice, dandelion, couch grass, aloe, and marshmallow.

MENOPAUSE Take dong quai, maca powder (regulates hormones), fish oil, black cohosh, flaxseed, probiotics, vitamins C and E, B-complex, red clover, valerian, ginseng, and evening primrose oil; avoid caffeine, chocolate, sugar and dairy; eat a balanced diet with greens, fruits, protein (less meat), seeds, and nuts.

MORNING SICKNESS Take Culing (a safe Chinese herb you can purchase online); eat protein frequently; maca powder, chamomile, rosemary, fennel, peppermint, ginger, licorice, and anise teas; take wild yam and catnip.

MOTION SICKNESS Eat ginger, soda crackers, fenugreek, fennel, rosemary, basil, cloves, licorice tea, peppermint, cinnamon, rosemary, horehound herb, valerian, chamomile, and catnip; get acupressure.

NOSEBLEED Take vitamins C, K, and E; take copper, iron, and zinc; rub vitamin E on nose; use cold compress; do not lie down (blood might go into throat); avoid aspirin and other blood thinners.

OILY SKIN Take omega-3 and flaxseed; avoid red meat, fried foods, and dairy products; use a cotton ball to dab face with neroli oil mixed with lavender; steam-clean face; dab on five drops of warm rosemary oil or apricot kernel oil; use a combination of yarrow, peppermint, and sage teas on face to remove oil; keep hands off face.

OSTEOPOROSIS Take vitamin D3 with calcium-rich foods (calcium supplements tend to create deposits, eat calcium-rich foods, instead); take manganese, DHEA, boron, chromium, and vitamins E and K2; eat dandelion, parsley, garlic, onions, kelp, turmeric, fenugreek, red clover, and cod liver oil.

PHOBIAS AND FEARS Soak in warm baths with lavender oil; get massages; exercise and do yoga; take valerian, hops, oatstraw, alfalfa, scullcap, passion flower, 5-HTP, melatonin, L-Theanine, verbena; vitamins C, D3, and B-complex; have doctor check your adrenal and thyroid levels; get acupressure or acupuncture to relieve stress; avoid caffeine, sugar, refined carbohydrates, sodas, dairy products, gluten, and wheat.

POISON OAK AND IVY Take homeopathic by Natra-Bio called Poison Ivy Poison Oak orally; apply black walnut tincture, bloodroot, echinacea, and goldenseal topically; use baking soda and water in bath; apply witch hazel to relieve itching and drying.

PMS Take dong quai, maca powder; white willow bark (for pain), burdock, St. John's wort, chasteberry, evening primrose oil, black cohosh, wild yam, ginkgo; chromium, magnesium, and vitamins D3, K2, and B6; use warm castor oil compresses on belly; take baths with lavender and Epsom salts.

RESTLESS LEG SYNDROME Take vitamin E, B-complex, D-ribose, iron, magnesium, St. John's wort; aconite, valerian, kava kava, hops, 5-HTP, and melatonin; drink oatstraw, chamomile, peppermint, or nettle tea; eat iron-rich foods; take warm lavender oil baths.

SHINGLES Avoid acidic foods and sugar; alkalize body with apple cider vinegar, cucumber, cabbage, aloe (topically or drink juice); licorice tea, ginseng, calendula (topically), use peppermint, oregano, rosemary, hyssop, thyme, and sage-- in tea or on food; take H-Plex Defense; avoid stress.

SORE THROAT Gargle with warm salt water; steam throat with eucalyptus oil; take goldenseal and echinacea tincture, colloidal silver, oregano oil, olive leaf extract, Yin Chiao (Chinese herb), isatis root tincture; vitamin C, and zinc lozenges.

STAINED TEETH Brush with baking soda and water, hydrogen peroxide, sage (boiled in water), charcoal, cuttlefish bone, myrrh; bay leaves in powder with orange peel poultice.

STRESS Take ashwagandha, lemon balm, licorice root, passion flower, 5-HTP, chamomile, oatstraw, and ginseng; drink lavender tea with hops and flaxseed, as well as lobelia, chamomile, and peppermint tea; engage in breathing techniques like yoga; meditate; do acupressure and acupuncture; take lavender oil baths.

TACHYCARDIA (Rapid Heartbeat) Take potassium (monitored by doctor), magnesium, L-carnitine, CoQ10; motherwort, goldenseal, cayenne pepper, valerian, arnica internally (homeopathic), black cohosh, hawthorn, ginseng, astragalus and ginkgo biloba; engage in deep breathing; drink relaxing teas; avoid sugar and dairy; **get medical evaluation.**

TENDONITIS Anti-inflammatory diet; take apple cider vinegar; stretch tendons gently; drink plenty of water; avoid acidic food;

take MSM, ginger, devil's claw, turmeric, boswellia, and bromelain to reduce inflammation; detoxify to eliminate toxins.

TOOTHACHE Use clove, peppermint, and oregano oils topically and orally; take white willow bark, colloidal silver, olive leaf extract, turmeric, and wheatgrass; detoxify bacteria; swish mouth with warm salt water.

ULCERS Avoid red meats, coffee, sugar, oranges, juice, dairy, alcohol, and acidic food; take ginger, dandelion, chicory, yellow dock, barberry, Oregon grape, gentian, mugwort; colloidal silver, oregano oil, olive leaf extract, isatis, andrographis, and probiotics.

VARICOSE VEINS Take bioflavonoids for circulation; take vitamins C, D3, K2, and E; take pycnogenol, magnesium, niacin; butcher's broom, grape seed, horse chestnut, gotu kola, and sweet clover; make topical use of anti-inflammation herbs such as a turmeric poultice; apply castor oil; avoid dairy, wheat, sugar, and alcohol.

WRINKLES Take antioxidants; take vitamins C, E, D3, and A; eat acai and mangosteen berries, and eggs; take moringa, hyaluronic acid, lysine, proline; chlorella, spirulina, omega, copper and zinc; grape-seed extract, aloe gel; use as poultice on face-- calendula oil, evening primrose oil, mullein, rose oil, and black seed salve.

HOME REMEDIES' WISDOM:

Use these remedies cautiously, unless you're familiar with them and feel comfortable. If you have questions, doubt, fear, concern or otherwise, consult a professional before practicing self-treatment. We all have different physical compositions, react differently to substances, and need to proceed in an informed and educated manner.

CHAPTER 10

RECIPES FOR HEALING

The following recipes are included because they all have healing properties for treating autoimmunity, and help keep the immune system clean and in balance.

Be mindful of buying local and organic products as much as possible, for adding value and healthy nutrition. If you're a savvy consumer and knowledgeable about foods, nutrition and cooking, you can vary ingredients according to taste, but try to maintain the integrity of the herbs and spices for the most desired effect. Always wash fruits and vegetables very well with an organic fruit/vegetable wash which you can purchase at Whole Foods or the supermarket.

DETOXIFICATION

These specific foods, herbs and spices are particularly effective for cleansing the body. They create delicious, cleansing and nutritious drinks and smoothies:

- Dandelion and beets clean liver.
- Greens clean and nourish cells.
- Lemons, apples, and ginger clean body.
- Cranberries clean bladder.
- Cucumbers and celery are natural diuretics.

ROARING ROOTS AND FRUIT FEAST

1 medium beet, steamed
4 carrots
1–2 parsnips
1 apple, cored
1 handful berries
1/2 garlic clove
1 tsp. finely ground ginger
1 tsp. ground cinnamon
1 cup lemon water

Combine ingredients in blender or juicer. Blend until smooth. Strain if necessary. Drink, or refrigerate for 1 day.

GREEN GARDEN JUICE

1 green apple
3 celery stalks
5 leaves of kale
1 handful of spinach
1 handful of parsley
1/2 garlic clove
Juice of 1 lime
Juice of 1 lemon
3 pieces of ginger
1/2 cup water

Combine ingredients in blender or juicer. Blend until smooth. Strain if necessary. Drink, or refrigerate for 1 day.

MORINGA MAGIC

1 cup blackberries
1 cup strawberries, hulled
1 cup blueberries
1 scoop moringa powder
3 pieces of ginger
1 tsp. cinnamon
Juice of 1 lemon with 1/2 cup water

Combine ingredients in blender. Blend until smooth. Strain if necessary. Drink, or refrigerate for 1 day.

BERRY BLUE

1 cup blueberries
1 cup blackberries
4 sprigs of dandelion greens
3 sprigs of mint leaves
3 pieces of ginger
3 tbsp. cooked rhubarb
1/2 cup water

Combine ingredients in blender. Blend until smooth. Strain if necessary. Drink, or refrigerate for 1 day.

V-10 MADNESS

1 peeled cucumber
2 carrots
1 tomato
2 stalks of celery

3 kale leaves
1 cup spinach
1 red pepper
2 sprigs of parsley
1/2 garlic clove
2 sprigs of basil
1/2 cup water

Combine ingredients in blender. Blend until smooth. Strain if necessary. Drink, or refrigerate for 1 day.

LEMON-GINGER SURPRISE

Juice of 1 lemon
2 stalks of asparagus (steamed)
3 large cauliflower pieces
2 carrots
1 apple, cored
3 pieces of ginger
2 sprigs of cilantro
1 tsp. maple syrup or honey
1 tsp. olive oil
1/3 cup water

Combine ingredients in blender. Blend until smooth. Strain if necessary. Drink, or refrigerate for 1 day.

SASSY SPIRULINA

4 spinach leaves
3 kale leaves
1 cooked beet

1 sweet potato
1 pinch cayenne pepper
1/2 garlic clove
1/2 tsp. cinnamon
2 sprigs of cilantro
1 tbsp. spirulina powder
1 tsp. chlorella powder
1/3 cup water

Combine ingredients in blender. Blend until smooth. Strain if necessary. Drink, or refrigerate for 1 day.

CUCUMBER CRUSH

3 pieces of ginger
1 sprig of mint
1-inch cut piece of fennel
1 radish
1/2 cucumber
1/2 apple, cored
1 stalk celery
1/4 cup water

Combine ingredients in blender. Blend until smooth. Strain if necessary. Drink, or refrigerate for 1 day.

The **MASTER CLEANSE** is a program that has been effective for many years. It's simple and detoxifying, and has three steps:

- Three days of gradually removing processed foods from diet.
- Three to ten days using ingredients in Master Cleanse to clean the body and lose weight. Do three days first and see

how you feel. Work up to ten days if you feel good and aren't having serious detoxification reactions.
- Three days after cleanse eating healthful foods again.
- Drink warm saltwater before bed (flushes toxins)

MASTER CLEANSE INGREDIENTS:

Juice of 1 lemon
Add 1 tbsp. maple syrup to 8 oz. water
1 pinch of cayenne pepper
6–10 glasses of water

Blend ingredients together. Put in container that is chemical-free. Sip the drink throughout the day with no food. You can drink water at any time. If you feel weak, nauseous or have a headache, flush more with water and stop drinking the Master Cleanse until symptoms lessen. Resume again when you feel more stable. If you feel good after three days, continue on with cleanse gradually for a maximum of ten days.

Check with your doctor or practitioner to make sure this cleanse is appropriate for you. If you've been diagnosed with candida, especially in elevated levels, do a different kind of cleanse that has no sugar or sweeteners.

VEGAN RECIPES

CURRY CRAZE

1 cup cooked basmati rice
2 cups cooked garbanzo or black beans

1 cup roasted Brussels sprouts or other greens
1 pinch cayenne pepper
1 tsp. ginger
1 tsp. cinnamon
1 to 2 tsp. curry powder
6 cloves garlic
3 tbsp. light soy sauce
1 tbsp. sesame oil
5 tbsp. olive oil
Raisins or currants, optional

Cook rice in 2 cups water for 20 minutes. In saucepan, brown garlic cloves in soy sauce, olive oil, and sesame oil on low to medium heat. Combine other ingredients, then sauté until blended and warm. Place cooked rice in bowl, add other ingredients, stir well, and serve. Add minimal raisins or currants if desired. Serves 2.

TEMPEH TRUIMPH

2 cups grilled, cubed tempeh
3 cups cauliflower
3 cups broccoli
1/2 cup slivered almonds
1/2 cup dried cranberries
1/2 cup sliced garlic cloves
1/2 cup chopped onions
1 tsp. curry powder
1 tsp. cumin
1 tsp. coriander
1/3 cup olive oil

Steam the vegetables. Saute onions and garlic in olive oil. Add spices, almonds, and cranberries. Gently mix in vegetables, and stir well. Heat to taste. Add pinch of salt and pepper. Serves 2.

FENNEL FANTASY

1 cup cooked red or white beans
2 cups cooked brown rice
1 fennel bulb, steamed and chopped
Juice of 1/2 lemon
1/4 cup dry white wine
1 tbsp. olive oil
1 tsp. dill
1 tsp. garlic powder
1 tsp. ginger
Pinch salt and pepper

Combine cooked beans and rice in skillet. Add white wine, olive oil, lemon juice, fennel, and spices. Heat for 15 minutes over medium to low heat. Stir, and serve. Serves 2 or 3.

SQUASH SYMPHONY

2 cups green and yellow squash, sliced
1 cup acorn squash, steamed, cut, and oven-roasted (with olive oil)
1 cup slivered cashews
1/2 cup goji berries or dried cranberries
1/3 cup sesame oil

1 tsp. molasses
1 tsp. tamari or light soy sauce
Juice of 1/2 lemon
3 tbsp. dry sherry
1 tsp. garlic powder
1 tsp. turmeric
1tsp. cardamom

Steam the green and yellow squash. In a skillet, combine roasted and cubed acorn squash with cashews, goji berries or cranberries, sesame oil, tamari, sherry, and molasses. Add lemon juice and spices, and cook over low to medium heat. Salt and pepper to taste. Serves 2.

ROCKIN' ROOTS

1 yellow beet, sliced
1 red beet, sliced
1 or 2 turnips, sliced
1 or 2 carrots, sliced
1 or 2 parsnips, sliced
1 cup cooked red lentils
2 sprigs mint
2 sprigs rosemary
5 tbsp. olive oil
2 tsp. sesame oil
1 onion
3 garlic cloves
1 tsp. turmeric
1 tsp. mustard powder
1 tsp. ginger

1 tsp. parsley
Pinch salt and pepper

Steam all sliced root vegetables until they are still a bit firm, and then roast vegetables with olive oil in oven for 20 minutes at 350 degrees. On stove in skillet with 5 tbsp. olive oil, brown garlic cloves. Add vegetables, spices, and herbs, and stir in 2 tsp. sesame oil. Cover, and heat on low for 15 minutes. Stir, and add salt and pepper. Serves 2.

PASTA PASSION

2 tbsp. extra-virgin olive oil
3 garlic cloves, browned in olive oil
2 cups artichoke hearts
1/4 cup pistachio nuts
3 tbsp. dried currants
1/4 tsp. Himalayan sea salt
1/4 tsp. ground black pepper
8 oz. pasta made from quinoa, cooked according to package instructions
3/4 cup fresh parsley, coarsely chopped
2 tbsp. red wine

Add garlic and olive oil to skillet, and heat over medium heat. Brown garlic, stirring until softened, about 5 minutes. Add artichoke hearts, pistachio nuts, and currants. Season with salt and pepper, and cook for 2 more minutes. Remove from heat. Add quinoa pasta to the skillet, and use tongs to toss well to combine. Add parsley and red wine, and heat for 2 minutes. Serves 2.

SOUPS FOR IMMUNITY

BONE BROTH BOOST

3 cups bone stock from chicken bones boiled and simmered in water for an hour on the stove
1 cup quinoa
1 clove garlic, grated
Juice of 1 lime or 1 lemon
1 tsp. dried fresh turmeric
3 tbsp. cold-pressed vegetable juice
1 pinch rosemary, cilantro, basil, parsley
1 small inch of fresh ginger root, grated
1 tsp. raw vegetables such as broccoli, kale, asparagus
1 cup fermented kimchi (optional)
1 tsp. apple cider vinegar or white wine
2 tbsp. olive oil
Pinch sea salt and freshly ground pepper

Cook quinoa by using bone stock instead of water (provides higher amounts of protein and flavor). Saute garlic in olive oil until brown. Add bone stock and white wine or apple cider vinegar. Cook, and stir occasionally until sauce is reduced by half. Add your favorite vegetable: broccoli, kale, asparagus and cook al dente (not overcooked). You may add 1 cup of fermented kimchi with vegetables, if desired.

YUMMY YAMS

6 small yams, skinned
3 cups vegetable broth

1 cup almond milk or coconut milk
1 tsp. curry powder
1 tsp. garlic powder
1 tsp. ground cinnamon
1 tsp. ground ginger
2 tbsp. coconut milk yogurt (optional)
Salt and pepper to taste

Boil broth in large saucepan. Add yams and spices; cover, and simmer until yams are tender. Drain yams, and blend in blender with 3 cups vegetable broth. Return to pan, add coconut milk, and simmer. Add salt and pepper, and a dollop of coconut milk yogurt if desired. Serves 2.

VIVACIOUS VEGETABLES

1 cup broccoli florets
1 cup sliced parsnips
1 cup cauliflower florets
4 cups chicken broth
3 sprigs mint
3 sprigs thyme
1 tsp. onion powder
1 tsp. nutmeg
1 tsp. coriander
Salt and pepper to taste

Steam broccoli and cauliflower florets, boil broth, and add all vegetables until tender. Add spices, and simmer for 20 to 25 minutes, then remove sprigs. Puree soup in blender until smooth. Return to saucepan, and simmer for 15 minutes. Serves 2.

CAGEY CABBAGE

1 head red cabbage, chopped
1 cup finely sliced tomatoes
6 cups water
1/3 cup Marsala wine
1 red pepper, chopped
3 carrots, sliced
3 celery stalks, sliced
1 onion, chopped
1 cup kale leaves, chopped
1 tsp. cilantro
1 tsp. thyme
1 tsp. sage
1 tsp. parsley
1 tsp. dill
Salt and pepper to taste

Boil water in large saucepan, and add all vegetables. Cook on medium heat, adding herbs, Marsala wine, and spices. Simmer for 20 to 25 minutes. Serves 2 or 3.

BASIL BLAST

2 cups cooked organic chicken breasts or tempeh, cubed
3 carrots, chopped
1 cup chopped spinach or chard
3 celery stalks, chopped
1 onion, chopped
4 cups chicken or vegetable stock

1 tbsp. coconut oil
2 tsp. holy basil
1 tsp. turmeric
2 garlic cloves, chopped
1 tsp. ground ginger
1 pinch cayenne pepper
1 tsp. thyme
Pinch of salt

Boil stock and add vegetables, coconut oil, onion, and cooked chicken or tempeh pieces. Add spices and herbs, cover, and simmer for 45 minutes, stirring occasionally. Serves 2 to 3.

COLD-CRUSHER

4 cups vegetable broth
4 garlic cloves
5 slices ginger root
1 tsp. cayenne pepper
1 tsp. curry powder
1 tsp. cumin
1 tsp. cinnamon
1 tsp. coriander
1 tsp. olive or coconut oil
Juice of 1 lemon
Pinch of salt

Add oil, lemon juice and spices to broth, boil, then simmer for 45 to 50 minutes. Serves 2 or 3.

CURRIED CARROT CRASHER

4 carrots, sliced
2 parsnips, sliced
2 celery stalks, sliced
2 sprigs parsley
1 tbsp. olive oil
1 cup water
1/3 cup grape-seed oil
1/8 cup lemon and lime juices
2 tsp. curry powder
1 tsp. turmeric
1 pinch cayenne pepper
1/3 cup brandy
1 tsp. garlic powder
1 tsp. cardamom
Pinch of salt

Steam all vegetables until soft, then put in large saucepan. Add water, oils, juices, brandy, herbs, and spices. Simmer for 45 minutes. Serves 2 to 3.

DELECTIBLE DESSERTS

BAKED APPLE ANTICS

1/2 cup almonds
1/2 cup cashews
1/2 cup organic cranberries
2 chopped figs

1 tsp. ginger
1 tsp. cinnamon
1/2 tsp. nutmeg
1/4 tsp. ground cloves
4 apples
1/4 cup honey or 6 drops of stevia
1 cup apple cider

Preheat oven to 325 degrees. Mix nuts or seeds, cranberries, figs, ginger root, and spices in a bowl. Don't peel the apples, since most of the fiber and nutrients are in the skin. **Stuff** each apple with the nut and seed mixture, then drizzle with honey and place in an 8-inch-by-8-inch square baking dish. Pour the juice around the fruit to keep it moist. Bake for 30 to 35 minutes, until fruit is soft. Serve warm. Serves 4.

KEY LIME LIMERICK

Crust

1 cup unsweetened shredded coconut
1 cup walnuts or almonds
1/4 tsp. Himalayan sea salt
1/2 cup pitted organic dates or figs

Filling

3 avocados
3 tbsp. lime juice
1 tsp. grated lime peel
1/2 cup raw honey or molasses
Pinch salt
Add fresh slices kiwi or lime fruit

Process coconut, walnuts or almonds, and salt in a food processor until coarsely ground. Add dates or figs, and process until the mixture begins to clump together. Press into the bottom and sides of a 9-inch pie plate. Place the crust in a freezer for 15 minutes. Process all filling ingredients in a food processor until smooth. **Pour** filling into the pie crust. Set in fridge for 20 minutes. Garnish with fresh slices of kiwi or lime fruit. Serves 4.

DARK CHOCO-CUPPIES
Cake

1 1/2 cups whole millet or quinoa pastry flour
1/3 cup unsweetened organic cocoa powder
1 tsp. baking soda
1/2 tsp. Himalayan sea salt
1 cup almond or coconut milk
3/4 cup sweet potato puree
1/4 cup (1/2 stick) unsalted butter or nondairy butter, room temperature
8 drops or 1/10 cup organic stevia
2 eggs
1 tsp. pure vanilla extract

Preheat oven to 375 degrees, and line a 12-cup muffin pan with paper liners. In a large bowl, whisk together flour, cocoa powder, baking soda, and salt. In a medium bowl, whisk together almond milk and sweet potato purée. With an electric mixer, cream together butter and sugar on high speed until light and fluffy. Add eggs and vanilla. Reduce speed to low, and add flour mixture in batches. Spoon batter into prepared muffin cups. Bake about 25 minutes, or until a toothpick inserted into the center of a cupcake comes out clean. Let cool in pan 10 minutes. Transfer to a wire rack to cool completely. When cooled, spread with glaze (recipe below). Makes 12 cupcakes.

Glaze

2 tsp. unsalted butter or nondairy butter
2 tbsp. almond or coconut milk
2 tbsp. cocoa powder
1 cup sifted powdered organic raw sugar or stevia powder
1/4 cup pecan or cashew pieces, coarsely chopped

Heat butter, milk, and cocoa in a small saucepan over medium heat, stirring until butter is melted and cocoa is dissolved. Transfer to a mixing bowl, and gradually whisk in organic sweetener. Let stand 15 minutes for glaze to thicken to spreading consistency. Spread over cupcakes, and top with nuts.

BANANA CHIP COOKIE-CRAZE

1 cup oat or hemp flour
3/4 cup steel-cut rolled oats
1/2 tsp. baking powder
1/3 tsp. baking soda
1/2 tsp. salt
1/2 cup raw sugar
1/3 cup grapeseed oil
1/3 cup plain almond or coconut milk
1/2 tsp. vanilla extract
1/2 ripe banana, cut into small pieces
1/4 cup chopped walnuts, cashews, or almonds
1/3 cup semisweet vegan chocolate chips

Preheat oven to 350 degrees. Combine first 6 ingredients in a bowl. Whisk together oil, almond milk, and vanilla in a separate bowl. Add wet mixture to dry ingredients; stir to combine. Add banana, nuts, and chocolate chips. Line a baking sheet with parchment paper, and scoop 1 inch pieces of dough into pan. Bake 25 minutes or until light brown, turning baking sheet halfway through. Let cool on a wire rack. Makes 12 cookies.

PUMPKIN-GINGERBREAD GALA

1/4 lb. canned pumpkin
Extra-virgin olive oil, for brushing
4 large eggs
1 cup packed brown raw sugar
1 1/2 tsp. ground cinnamon
1/4 tsp. ground nutmeg
1/4 tsp. ground allspice
2 cups coconut milk cream
1 1/2 tsp. pure vanilla extract
1 loaf cinnamon or plain pound cake, diced
1/2 cup golden raisins, currants, goji berries, or cranberries
1/4 cup diced crystallized ginger

Preheat oven to 375 degrees. In a large bowl, combine 2 1/2 cups of the pumpkin puree, eggs, brown sugar, and spices. Whisk in coconut cream and vanilla. Combine cake, raisins, and ginger in a 7-inch-by-11-inch baking dish. Pour pudding mixture over bread to cover, and let sit 15 minutes. Bake in preheated oven until custard is set, about 40 minutes. Serves 4.

These recipes are designed to support immunity, healing and joy! They are delicious, nutritious and fun to make. They are only a small number of healthful and immune-building recipes available, and for those of you who like to be creative, you can create your own combinations, using ingredients that you favor.

This book is your guide to immunity and autoimmune disorders, including cancer. And these recipes are a special added attraction. Use the information as a guide to knowledge, information, education, and most of all, hope for your health, both for now and the future!

EPILOGUE

THE FUTURE OF YOUR HEALTH

I have witnessed an impressive number of people healing from a variety of diseases in different stages, including my own. As you gleaned from reading this book, holistic healing, which means body/mind/spirit connectivity, is possible under the appropriate professional guidance and with the support of loved ones and friends.

We are on the cutting edge of a new paradigm in medicine and holistic, natural health. As I mentioned before, several medical schools are now offering courses in integrative, functional medicine, which means that medical doctors are now being trained to treat core or root issues in healing. That is the essence of functional medicine – to reach the root problem with whatever natural means are available and appropriate, and work from the inside to the outside of the body. This includes the use of the spiritual, physical and emotional practices, which are discussed in the book.

There is an "attitude of healing" that accompanies wellness. Utilizing the tools of healing such as meditation, yoga, deep and conscious breathing techniques, talking with therapists or counselors when indicated, creative visualization, support groups and positive mental conditioning, are mandated for significant and lasting healing.

You read the stories in the book of people who were cured from pathogenic illnesses and disorders, including those of the mind.

In fact, as you may have learned, more often than not, mental illness is increased from disturbances with the gut microbiome.

By identifying the underlying cause of almost all disease, we're able to address the issue with effective treatment.

By the same token, what are the effects of genetics and DNA on health, and can we reverse these indicators and by-pass heredity? We believe we can; there is strong scientific evidence available which corroborates that nutritional practices and attitude/lifestyle, along with herbs, supplements and uncommon protocols, can literally alter DNA. Just because your mother has the gene for breast cancer and you do, too, doesn't preclude that you'll develop breast cancer.

We're also greatly affected by environmental factors, and there is a call to action for us to participate in getting laws passed that limit pollution from industry and its effect on consumer products, including foods.

We're experiencing global transformation on many levels, and the future is both exciting and promising, and needs our help and participation. We hold the key to our own lives, and I urge you to join the revolution and advocate for your health and welfare.

Naturally, there are those who will want to defend the existing paradigm, but science tells us that we're now on the forefront of remarkable and rewarding possibilities for change. We have the opportunity to take back both our health and our world, through all of the measures recommended in this book. Let's begin our journey now; there is no better time than the present!

AUTHOR'S NOTE

I hope you all gained insight, information, knowledge, understanding, and hope from reading this book. It's been a long, passionate, and exhilarating journey on my part, and my intention is always to help and heal you.

We are an extremely complex species, with an infinite number of energetic components, variables, genetics, and beliefs. Every part of us informs every other part, and it's an extraordinarily fascinating, synergistic holograph.

"Holistic health" incorporates those parts of us in a functioning totality. Knowledge empowers us to make healthful choices for our body/mind/spirit connection.

This book offers you the tools. Because I, personally, have been on both sides of the health spectrum—the healed and the healer—I understand how it all comes together. I don't always "do it right," believe me, but I do know what is right and what isn't.

My wish is that you are all inspired to make healthful decisions based on accurate information. Know that we are all children of the same God—we have the power to love, forgive, embrace, surrender, receive, accept, be authentic and playful, inspire, inform, and give back to those who need our help.

Thank you for sharing this with me, and may we all keep loving and learning on this journey of life.

Love, Blessings, and Optimum Wellness

GLOSSARY

A

Acai berry—promotes weight loss; anti-aging and antioxidant

Acesulfame K—sugar substitute, highly toxic to kidneys and organs

Acetylcysteine—protects against pulmonary diseases

Acetylglucosamine—anti-inflammatory for osteoarthritis, IBS, and Crohn's

Acetylneuraminic acid—derivative of sugar

Acrylamide—neurotoxin affects brain and nervous system

Adaptogen—helps body adapt to stress

Adenine—functional component of DNA

Agrimony—herb for relieving excess grief and sadness

AGS, Glycoside—sugar component

Aloe vera juice—helps support digestive function

Alpha lipoic acid—helps neuropathy, brain function, and aging

Aluminum—chemical element, metal

Alzheimer's—loss of brain function as brain shrinks, dementia

Ammonia—gas that is poisonous if inhaled, gives off toxic vapors

Amyotrophic lateral sclerosis—degenerative neurological condition that affects the whole body

Anemia—body does not have enough healthy red blood cells

Angelica—herb good for colds, coughs, sinuses, and urinary tract

Antigenic—stimulates production of antibodies against toxins, bacteria, and foreign blood cells

Angiogenesis—process by which tumors set up their own blood supply

Antimony—chemical element and metalloid in nature

Antioxidants—molecules that protect the cells against toxins, help fight infection and diseases

Apoptosis—programmed cell death

Arginine—amino acid for heart health, supports blood and oxygen flow, helps body make proteins

Arsenic—toxic chemical element

Arthritis—inflammation of the joints

Ashwagandha—Ayurvedic herb for stress, anxiety, and depression

Aspartame—artificial sweetener, turns to formaldehyde in body, toxic to nervous system

Autism—developmental disorder that appears within the first three years of life, affects normal brain development of social skills

Autoimmune disease—failure of organism to recognize its parts, immune response against its cells and tissues

Ayurvedic—Indian traditional medicine, holistic

B

Bacopa—herb good for memory, Alzheimer's, anxiety, ADHD, epilepsy, and joint pain

Bacteria—large family of microorganisms

BHA/BHT—preservatives added to foods to prevent fat spoilage

Bentonite—detoxification clay, makes body pH more alkaline

Betaine hydrochloride—organic compound supports protein digestion and gastric pH balance; enhances calcium, iron, and B12

Biohazards—biological hazards, as in chemical warfare

Black cohosh—helps with hot flashes from menopause and hormone imbalance

Black walnut—herb for anti-inflammatory against harmful organisms and parasites, supports digestion and blood detoxification

Bladderwrack—seaweed used for underactive thyroid, goiter, iodine digestive disorders, blood cleansing, and immunity

B-lymphocytes—essential to immunity, produced in bone marrow and white blood cells

Boswellia—Ayurvedic herb useful for reducing inflammation

Bromelain—extract from stems of pineapple, reduces inflammation

Bruxism—teeth grinding

Bupleurum—Chinese herb for treating respiratory infections, flu, pneumonia, and hepatitis C

Bursitis—swelling of the sac that cushions muscles, tendons, and joints

C

Cadmium—chemical hazard in water, toxic

Calendula—plant remedy for healing cuts and other minor skin injuries

Candida—the most common fungal infection, overload might cause serious autoimmune disorders

Caprylic acid—natural antifungal for treating candida

Capsicum—from a nightshade plant for helping digestion, heart, and blood, and reducing inflammation

Carbaryl—pesticide that is poisonous to humans and animals

Carcinogens—substances that cause cancer

Cayenne—spice that helps sore throat, stimulates circulation, helps high blood pressure

Cardamom—spice in ginger family that aids with digestion, detoxification, colds, flu, cancer, blood pressure, anti-inflammation

Carpal tunnel syndrome—pressure on median nerve in wrist, can cause tingling or weakness and muscle damage

Cellulite—pockets of fat with toxins, looks like ripples

Chamomile—herb that calms anxiety and soothes stomach

Chasteberry—fruit from an herb good for PMS, menopause, and infertility; controls bleeding; increases breast milk

Chelation therapy—administration of chelating elements to remove heavy metals from the body

Chemical trails—"chemtrails" are toxic substances dropped from planes; used to experiment with weather patterns; developed by multinational agricultural biotech corporations; very toxic to the earth, humans, and animals

Chlordane—man-made pesticide toxic to organisms

Chlorinated aliphatic hydrocarbons—toxic chlorinated solvents in ground water and soil

Choline—substance made in liver; good for treating memory loss, seizures, and brain disorders

Crohn's disease—deep inflammation of the bowel, causing diarrhea, pain, blood in stool, and gastrointestinal distress

Chronic fatigue syndrome—virus that causes extreme fatigue, depression, and muscle aches

Cinnamon bark—balances blood sugar, diabetes, and colds; soothes upset stomach.

Citrus seed extract—treats fungus, bacteria, and virus

Colloidal silver—mineral that treats fungus, virus, bacteria, pneumonia, flu, and Lyme disease (viral)

CoQ10—part of the chain of chemical reactions that creates energy within cells

Cortisol—stress hormone

Cryptosporidium—giardia, parasites in intestines of humans and animals

Cystic fibrosis—autoimmune disorder that causes mucus in lungs and other organs

Cysteine—amino acid that is a building block for proteins, used to prevent certain diseases

Cytokines—chemical messengers that trigger normal cells to grow and repair

Cytomegalovirus—virus from chickenpox, herpes family

D

Dandelion—diuretic; lowers blood pressure; cleans liver, kidneys, and gallstones; aids digestion

Dong quai—tones blood, regulates menstruation and hormones, moistens, reduces palpitations, reduces swelling

Dengue fever—infectious tropical disease caused by virus; causes fever, joint pain, headache, and skin rash

Dermatitis—skin inflammation caused by fungus, dry skin, or allergy

Devil's claw—herb that is anti-inflammatory, good for appetite, reduces cholesterol

DHEA—hormone made by human body, helps sugar metabolism and adrenal fatigue

Diabetes—high blood sugar, pancreas not producing enough insulin or cells do not respond to insulin, frequent urination and unquenchable thirst

Diacetyl—chemical in artificial butter

Dichlorophene—pesticide toxic to many organisms

Diethylene glycol—colorless flammable gas, toxic to organisms

Diflucan—drug that treats fungal infection, candida

Dinucleotide NADH—coenzyme in all cells, helps oxidation and glucose/energy metabolism

Diverticulosis—pouches form in walls of the intestines, caused by not chewing foods well

DNA—heredity material of all genes and organisms

Dupuytren's contracture—autoimmune disorder caused from toxins, tissues of hands and feet contract to form rope-like cords and stiffness

E

Echinacea—herb from a flowering plant, which is good for colds, sore throat, flu, swollen glands, and immune system

Eczema—atopic dermatitis causes dryness, itching, redness, and irritation

Elderberry—flowering plant that treats colds, flu, immunity, sinuses, bronchitis, diabetes, red eyes, and joint pain

Emphysema—lung disease in which air sacs in the lungs cause difficulty in breathing

Endometriosis—cells in the uterus grow in other areas of the body, causing bleeding, pain, and infertility

Epstein-Barr virus—virus from the chickenpox and/or herpes family, which might cause extreme fatigue, swollen glands, lethargy, depression, and weakening of the immune system

Essiac tea—herbal tea that helps treat cancer and other illnesses; a combination of the herbs burdock root, sheep sorrel, slippery elm, and rhubarb root

Ethylenediamine—tetra-acetic acid that is toxic to humans

Ethylene glycol—toxic chemical found in many household products, might cause harm to humans

Esters—chemical compounds that react with water to produce alcohols and acids

Evening primrose oil—treats eczema, psoriasis, arthritis, multiple sclerosis, cancer, high cholesterol, and heart disease

F

Fenugreek—herb that might treat stomach inflammation, cholesterol, kidneys, and cancer

Feverfew—herb that might prevent headaches, migraines, dizziness, nausea, allergies, and asthma

Fibromyalgia—autoimmune disorder that might cause painful joints and muscles, inflammation, fatigue, headaches, depression, and anxiety

Fluoride—inorganic chemical; main component of fluorite, which might be harmful to humans

Formaldehyde—organic chemical that might be toxic to humans

Fracking—water mixed with sand and chemicals and injected at high pressure to create fractures in the earth, causing ground water to become toxic

Fucoidan—element in brown seaweed, used to treat cancer and other diseases

Fungus—organisms such as yeast, molds, and mushrooms

G

GABA—chemical made in brain, relieves anxiety and PMS, might stabilize blood pressure

Galactosemia—disorder that affects one's ability to metabolize sugar

Ganoderma—species of mushroom that might help combat virus, insomnia, stomach, bronchitis, flu, lungs, and immune system

Gentian root—helps digestion, liver tonic and anti-inflammatory

Germanium—chemical element that might help heart and blood vessels, glaucoma, and liver conditions

Ginger root or powder—alleviates nausea, food poisoning, morning sickness, and inflammation; boosts immunity

Ginkgo biloba—herb that improves blood flow to brain, might help memory and circulation

Goldenseal—herb might help colds, flu, sore throat, ulcers, colitis, and diarrhea

Ginseng—increases stamina; an adaptogen; helps hepatitis C menopause, glucose levels, cholesterol, and antiaging

Glutamine—most abundant amino acid in the body, building block of protein, helps build muscle mass, supports intestinal tract and pH balance in the body

Glutathione—most important antioxidant molecule, which might help cancer, autism, and other immune disorders

Gluten—protein composite found in foods processed with wheat and grains

GMO—genetically modified foods produced from the seeds of GMO organisms in crops, might affect human and animal organ function

Grape seed extract—derivatives of grape seeds, which have a high concentration of Vitamin E; might improve circulation, eyesight, cholesterol, and diabetes; protects cell damage; anti-inflammatory

Green tea—antioxidant, antiviral, antibacterial, and immune-boosting

H

Hawthorn berries—herbs that might be good for heart, circulation, blood vessels, and cholesterol

Heavy metals—metals such as mercury, cadmium, aluminum, antimony, and arsenic, which might cause health problems in humans

Herbicides—chemicals used to manipulate undesirable vegetation, might be harmful to humans

Herpes—virus from the chickenpox family that causes painful blisters and swelling

Holistic—understanding and consideration of the parts in relationship to the whole

Homeopathics—cell salts that might help the body's system heal itself

Honokiol—compound from the magnolia officinalis tree, used to treat cancer and immunity

Hormones—the body's natural chemical messengers

Hops—herb from a plant that might help sleep, anxiety, nerves, attention deficit disorder, indigestion, tuberculosis, and bladder infections

H. pylori—bacterial infection that might cause bloating, nausea, vomiting, and abdominal discomfort

Hydrochloric acid—toxins that might cause gastritis, bronchitis, and dermatitis

Hydroxide—hydrogen and oxygen form salts

Hypothyroidism—thyroid gland does not make enough thyroid hormone, might cause numerous symptoms and disease

I

Immunity—everything that relates to the immune system and its functions

Immunocytes—cells of lymph glands that might help immune functions and maturation of **B** cells

Inflammation—biological response to harmful stimuli, one component of all disease

Inositol—substance found in plants that might help nerve pain, panic, depression, cancer, psoriasis, autism, and cholesterol

Interferon alpha—naturally occurring proteins that might treat viral infections and immunity

IP6—cyclic acid that might be effective for cancer treatment, repairs gene mutations, establishes cellular communication

Irritable Bowel Syndrome—autoimmune disorder that might cause bowel inflammation, diarrhea or constipation, pain, and bloating in the stomach and intestines

Isatis root—herb that might help treat colds, flu, viruses, and bacteria

K

Kava kava—herb that relieves stress; helps sleep; treats anxiety; acts as an antifungal, antispasmodic, diuretic, and tranquilizer

Ketones—organic compound produced when body burns fat for energy or fuel

Kudzu vine—helps reduce cravings for alcohol; treats headaches, dizziness, aids circulation, blood pressure, and sinus infections

L

Lead—chemical element that is soft and malleable, toxic in high exposures

Licorice root—might help with digestion, chronic fatigue, ulcers, food poisoning, lupus, and inflammation; balances other herbs in combination

Linoleic Acid—substance that might fight cancer, hardening of the arteries, and obesity; helps immunity; aids weight loss

Lomatium root—broad-spectrum herb for antiviral, antibacterial, upper-respiratory, and anti-inflammatory treatment

Lupus—autoimmune disorder that might cause chronic inflammation, kidney failure, rash, joint and muscle pain, headaches, and a range of other symptoms

Lycium berries—also called wolfberries or goji berries, which might enhance immunity, liver function, eyesight, and circulation

Lyme disease—disease caused from a deer tick, which creates an infectious bacteria; early symptoms are flu-like feeling, fever, headaches, rash, and swollen lymph nodes

Lymphatic System—network of organs and lymph nodes, helps rid body of toxins, moves lymphatic fluid through tissues and bloodstream

M

Magnesium—key mineral in human metabolism; might be good for heart, muscles and tendons, kidneys, and detoxification of heavy metals

Mangosteen—fruit that might benefit the immune system; helps treat diarrhea, urinary tract infection, arthritis, cancer, and mental health

Mannose—sugar molecule important in human metabolism of proteins

Mercury—toxic chemical element liquid found in burning coal, light bulbs, batteries, and fish; harmful to humans

Methanol—wood alcohol produced from carbon methyl hydroxide

Microbes—single-cell organisms and the oldest form of life

Milk thistle—herb known to lower cholesterol and clean liver, benefits diabetes, has antioxidant and anti-inflammatory benefits

Modified citrus pectin—also known as PectaSol, might have numerous cancer-fighting and cardiovascular benefits

Molybdenum—metallic substance, cofactor of enzymes, aids in metabolism of fat and carbohydrates

Morinda root—herb that might help kidney, gallbladder, cancer, and urinary tract

Multiple sclerosis—autoimmune disorder often caused from candida, disrupts the myelin sheath in the brain and causes neurological problems in the immune system

Mycotoxins—secondary metabolites produced by micro-fungi, might cause serious illness in humans and animals

N

Neroli oil—nontoxic oil relieves tension and anxiety, helps circulation

Neurotoxins—chemicals that damage brain and nervous system by killing neurons

Niacin—vitamin B3, balances cholesterol and triglycerides, helps circulation and arteries

Nitrates—substance used in preserving meats, thought to be harmful in humans

NK Cells—white blood cells that help protect against viruses and cancer

Nystatin—plant-based substance for treating candida overgrowth and fungus

O

Oatstraw—herb that might help increase circulation, alleviate joint pain, and treat blood pressure problems, cancer, ulcers, and stomach cramps

Olestra—fat substitute that depletes blood levels of valuable fat-soluble substances

Olive leaf extract—contains phenols, which fight infections, viruses, fungus, inflammation, and tumors, and might balance blood pressure

Oregano oil—treats parasites, viruses, bacterial infections, allergies, sinus infections, colds, flu, earaches, and skin problems

Oregon grape root-—herb used to treat ulcers, stomach problems, and bowel infections (fungal and bacterial)

P

Palliative—focuses on relieving and preventing suffering

Parkinson's disease—autoimmune disorder of the brain that affects the nervous system, some research suggests it comes from toxins in the environment

Passion flower—flowering plant used to relieve insomnia, stomach upset, anxiety, seizures, asthma, palpitations, and pain

Pau d'Arco—herb used to treat cancer, candida, diabetes, and lupus; is anti-inflammatory

Perchlorate—salts that occur naturally and are man-made, contaminate ground water

Perchlorethylene—chemical used in dry cleaning, prolonged use might affect lungs and skin

PEG-80—sorbitan laurate, chemical found in cosmetics

PFOA or C8—synthetic carboxylic acid, toxic man-made substance for nonstick cookware

Pinellia—drying herb; good for nausea, morning sickness, flu, and vomiting

Pituitary gland—small pea-size gland that releases hormones; affects growth, sexual development, metabolism, and reproduction

Potassium bromate—food additive linked to cancer

Propolis—from bee pollen; treats cancer, sores, allergies, throat, and ulcers; antioxidant and anti-inflammatory

Poly-MVA—liquid supplement to support cellular energy production

Probiotics—small organisms that help maintain natural flora in intestines

Protocols—a system of rules or procedures

Psoriasis—skin condition that causes flaky red scales, itching, inflammation, and irritation

Pulsatilla—clears and detoxifies poisons, antibacterial

Pycnogenol—from pine bark; used to treat female reproductive issues, heart, blood vessels, diabetes, ADHD, digestive problems, circulation, immune response, inflammation, respiratory health, and erectile dysfunction

R

Red clover—herb that treats immune system, blood congestion, and menopause; has valuable nutrients

Radix rehmanniae—herb used to treat blood loss and yin deficiency

Rhubarb—good source of fiber, polyphenols, minerals, antioxidant, B-complex vitamins, vitamin K, and amino acids

RNA—large biological molecules that perform vital roles in coding, decoding, and regulating expression of genes

S

Senna—herb that treats constipation, irritable bowel syndrome, and hemorrhoids, and balances weight

Shisandra—herbal adaptogen; regulates blood sugar and blood pressure, cholesterol, asthma, sleep, liver disease, and night sweats

Scullcap—herb treats nervous system, sleep disorders, well-being, and relaxation

Slippery elm bark—herb for treating sore throats, irritable bowel, bladder and urinary tract infections, colitis, diverticulitis, gout, and cold sores

Sodium hypochlorate—disinfectant that might adversely affect throat and stomach, and cause coughing

Spirulina—superfood, plant protein; might be good for treating allergies, immune system, blood pressure, cholesterol, and cancer

Succimer—a white crystalline powder that is a heavy metal detoxifier

Sulfites—chemicals used as a preservative to prevent discoloration in foods

T

T-cells—type of red blood cells central to immunity

Theanine—amino acid that might help anxiety, blood pressure, and Alzheimer's disease

Thermography—infrared imaging of breasts and entire body

Thyroid—one of the largest endocrine glands, produces hormones

Toxins—poisonous substances produced in living cells, might cause disease

Trichloromethane—also known as chloroform, health hazard, volatile liquid once used an anesthetic

Tryptophan—amino acid that regulates appetite, promotes sleep, treats anxiety and depression, and elevates mood

Turmeric—spice that supports immunity and liver function, and is anti-inflammatory

Tyrosine—amino acid that alleviates effects of stress and dopamine in brain, might be good for treating depression

V

Valerian—herb used to calm anxiety and panic attacks, promotes sleep and relaxation

W

White willow bark—alleviates pain, headaches, muscle soreness, and arthritis, and lowers fever

X

Xylitol—sugar substitute

Xylose—white crystalline sugar

Y

Yarrow—herb that treats bleeding ulcers, colds, hemorrhoids, bloating, and internal bleeding

Yin Chiao—herb that supports immune system; circulates lungs; treats headaches, flu, colds, cough, sore throat, angina, and fever

ABOUT THE AUTHOR

Sarah Zitin is a Certified Holistic Practitioner specializing in Chinese herbs, nutrition, supplements, and uncommon protocols for healing autoimmune disorders. She has been in practice for twenty years and has an innate, intuitive, and unique ability to assess and evaluate illness in the body. Her specialty is immunity and autoimmune disorders, and she has been successfully treating clients for many years.

Sarah studied at the School of Chinese Herbology in Berkeley, California. She has completed workshops at the Jaffe Institute of Medical and Spiritual Healing in Napa Valley, and Every Woman's Village in Los Angeles, and continues to study, evaluate, and observe the effects of nutrition, herbs, vitamins, and supplements on the body. Sarah has published various articles in magazines, journals, and online on holistic, integrative, and alternative health.

Sarah is an author and has a private practice in Studio City, California.

BIBLIOGRAPHY

GLUTATHIONE

Sechi G, Deledda MG, Bua G, Satta WM, Deiana GA, Pes GM, Rosati G. "Reduced intravenous glutathione in the treatment of early Parkinson's disease," *Prog Neuropsychopharmacol Biol Psychiatry Journal* 1996 Oct; 20(7):1159–70

Dalhoff K, Ranek L, Mantoni M, Poulsen, HE. "Glutathione treatment of hepatocellular carcinoma," *Liver* 1992; 12:341–343

Novi AM. "Regression of aflatoxin B1-induced hepatocellular carcinomas by reduced glutathione," *Science* 1981; 212:541–542

Kidd PM. "Glutathione: systemic protectant against oxidative and free radical damage," *Altern Med Rev* 1997; 2:155–176

HONOKIOL

JW Chen JT, Hong CY. "Honokiol traverses the blood-brain barrier and induces apoptosis of neuroblastoma cells via an intrinsic bax-mitochondrion-cytochrome c-caspase protease pathway," *Neuro Oncol.* 2012; 14(3):302–314

Xu D, Lu Q, Hu X. "Down-regulation of P-glycoprotein expression in MDR breast cancer cell MCF-7/ADR by honokiol," *Cancer Lett* 2006; 243(2):274–280

Wang X, Duan X, Yang G, et al. "Honokiol crosses BBB and BCSFB, and inhibits brain tumor growth in rat 9L intracerebral gliosarcoma model and human U251 xenograft glioma model," *PLoS One.* 2011; 6(4):e18490. doi: 10.1371/journal.pone.0018490

Xu HL, Tang W, Du GH, Kokudo N. "Targeting apoptosis pathways in cancer with magnolol and honokiol, bioactive constituents of the bark of Magnolia officinalis," *Drug Discov Ther.* 2011; 5(5):202–10

Arora S, Bhardwaj A, Srivastava SK, et al. "Honokiol arrests cell cycle, induces apoptosis, and potentiates the cytotoxic effect of gemcitabine in human pancreatic cancer cells," *PLoS One.* 2011; 6(6): e21573

Singh T, Prasad R, Katiyar SK. "Inhibition of class 1 histone deacetylases in non-small cell lung cancer by honokiol leads to suppression of cancer cell growth and induction of cell death in vitro and in vivo," *Epigenetics.* 2013; 8(1):54–65

IP6

Dr. Kin Vanderlinden, Dr. Ivana Vucenik, journals "Too Good to be True?"

Dr. Abulkalam Shamsuddin, based on studied research, "IP6 Natural Revolutionary Cancer Fighter"

POLY-MVA

NOTE: Before Poly-MVA, Dr. Josef Issels, the father of alternative medicine in Germany, reported 18.5 percent of terminal patients he treated lived five years or longer. Many alternative physicians in the United States are achieving similar results. Issels's treatments were health-supporting as opposed to current cancer-destructive methods. Our use with Poly-MVA has been limited to three years. In almost all cancers where the product was used, patients reported improvement of symptoms. More studies are necessary to assess the extent it prolongs life. Poly-MVA can be used as an adjuvant to cancer-destruction methods with great benefit to the patient—but for best results, it is used with other health-supporting regimens.

(rHS) Measurement of the Biological Terrain by Robert C. Greenberg. TLfDP Aug-Sept 1997. P. 64–68, article published in *Biomedical Therapy, 1998*

GERMANIUM

Clinical Trials.gov. Use of Organic Germanium or Placebo for the Prevention of Radiation Induced Fatigue. Accessed at www.clinicaltrials.gov/ct2/show/NCT00651417term=germanium&rank=1 on July 26, 2011

Food Standards Agency (UK), Expert Group on Vitamins and Minerals. Risk assessment: germanium, 2003. Accessed at www.food.gov.uk/multimedia/pdfs/evm_germanium.pdf on July 25, 2011

Gerber GB, Leonard A. "Mutagenicity, carcinogenicity and teratogenicity of germanium compounds," *Mutat Res.* 1997; 387:141-146

Lück BE, Mann H, Melzer H, Dunemann L, Begerow J. "Renal and other organ failure caused by germanium intoxication," *Nephrol Dial Transplant.* 1999 Oct; 14(10):2464–2468

Memorial Sloan-Kettering Cancer Center. Germanium. Accessed at www.mskcc.org/mskcc/html/69232.cfm on July 25, 2011.

National Products Association. Germanium. Accessed at www. naturalproductsassoc.org/site/PageServer?pagename=rr_bg_germanium on June 4, 2008. Content no longer available.

PDRhealth. Germanium. Accessed at www.pdrhealth.com/drug_info/nmdrugprofiles/nutsupdrugs/ger_0119.shtml on June 4, 2008. Content no longer available.

Schauss AG. "Nephrotoxicity and neurotoxicity in humans from organogermanium compounds and germanium dioxide," *Biol Trace Elem Res.* 1991 Jun; 29(3):267–280

Tao SH, Bolger PM. "Hazard assessment of germanium supplements," *Regul Toxicol Pharmacol.* 1997; 25:211–219

US Food and Drug Administration. Import Alert #54-07, Germanium Products, 3/18/11. Accessed at www.accessdata.fda.gov/cms_ia/importalert_139.html on July 25, 2011

US Food and Drug Administration. Memorandum in response to new dietary ingredient notification, November 13, 2002. Accessed at www.fda.gov/ohrms/DOCKETS/dockets/95s0316/95s-0316-rpt0155-01-vol113.pdf on July 25, 2011

MODIFIED CITRUS PECTIN

Jiang J, Eliaz I, Sliva D. "Synergistic and additive effects of modified citrus pectin with two polybotanical compounds, in the suppression of invasive behavior of human breast and prostate cancer cells," *Integr Cancer Ther.* 2013 Mar; 12(2):145–52

AGS-GLYCOSIDE COMPONENT

Chen, J. et al. Research on the antitumor effect of ginsenoside Rg3 in B16 melanoma cells. Melanoma Res. 2008 Oct; 18(5):322-9. Retrieved from http://www.ncbi.nlm.nih.gov/pubmed/18781130 Jia, W. "What is sapogenin?" Dammarane Sapogenin website. Retrieved from http://www.sapogenin.info/

FUCOIDAN

Bradley J. Wilcox, M.D., D. Craig Willcox, Ph.D., and Makoto Suzuki, M.D. *The Okinawa Diet Plan Get Leaner, Live Longer, and Never Feel Hungry,* Clarkson Potter/Publishers, New York, 2004. Jacket cover.

Hirayasu H, et al. "Sulfated polysaccharides derived from dietary seaweeds increase the esterase activity of a lymphocyte tryptase, granzyme A," *J Nutr Sci Vitaminol* (Tokyo). 2005 Dec:51(6):475–7

Giraux J., et al. "Modulation of human endothelial cell proliferation and migration by fucoidan and heparin," *Eur J Cell Biol* 1998 Dec; 77(4):352–9

Van Oosten M, et al. "Scavenger receptor-like receptors for the binding of lipopolysaccharide and lipoteichoic acid to liver endothelial and Kupffer cells," *J Endotoxin Res* 2001; 7(5):381–4

Thorlacius H, et al. "The polysaccharide fucoidan inhibits microvascular thrombus formation from P- and L-selection in vivo," *E Jour Clin Invest* 2000 Sept; 30(9):804–10

7 Ryan Drum, "Medical Uses of Seaweeds," http://ryandrum.com/seaweeds.htm

COLLOIDAL SILVER

http://curezone.com/foods/silver.asp
http://www.saltlakemetals.com/Silver_Antibacterial.htm
http://www.whale.to/a/robey1.html
http://health.centreforce.com/health/silver.html
http://www.naturalnews.com/038579_colloidal_silver_healing_water.html#ixzz2Wmq7TLqj

ONLINE STORES FOR HERBS, SUPPLEMENTS AND NUTRITION

Agelessherbs.com
A1supplements.com
Azurestandard.com

Bluedragonherbs.com
Botanicchoice.com

Chineseherbsdirect.com

Econugenics.com
Enzymatictherapy.com
Ez-healthsolutions.com

Healeo.com
Heavenandherbs.com
Herbalremedies.com
Herbspro.com
Howfoods.com

iHerb.com

Livingearthherbs.com
Localharvest.org

Newchapter.com
Nutricology.com
Nutritionexpress.com

Oregonswildharvest.com
Organickingdom.com

Standard process.com

Thenaturalonline.com
Thesynergycompany.com
Tibetanherbs.com
Truefoodsmarket.com

Vibranthealth.us
Vegancuts.com
Vitacost.com
Vitaminworld.com